Micrographia Restaurata

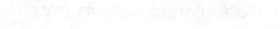

MICROGRAPHIA RESTAURATA:

OR, THE

COPPER-PLATES

OF

Dr. *HOOKE*'s Wonderful Difcoveries

BY THE

MICROSCOPE,

Reprinted and fully Explained:

Whereby the moft Valuable PARTICULARS in that

Celebrated AUTHOR's

MICROGRAPHIA

Are brought together in a narrow Compafs ;

AND

Intermixed, occafionally, with many Entertaining and Inftructive DISCO-
VERIES and OBSERVATIONS in NATURAL HISTORY.

Rerum Natura nufquam magis quàm in minimis tota eft.
PLIN. Hift. Nat. Lib. XI. C. 2.

LONDON.

Printed for and Sold by JOHN BOWLES, Printfeller at the *Black Horfe* in *Cornhill*.
Sold alfo by R. DODSLEY, in *Pallmall*, and JOHN CUFF, Optician, in *Fleetftreet*.
MDCCXLV.

THE

PREFACE.

THE MICROGRAPHIA of Dr. HOOKE being grown extremely scarce, and the Price thereof greatly raised; it can fall into the Hands of very few who are not so lucky to be possessed of it already; which (since a Desire of searching into the minute Wonders of Nature is become almost general) must be looked on as a great Misfortune, by many, who would gladly inform themselves what Discoveries were made by this *industrious Observer*, at a Time when *Microscopes* were very rare, and the Use of them but little known.

This Misfortune may, 'tis hoped, be however considerably alleviated, by a fortunate Preservation of nearly all the *Copper-Plates*, which the Doctor, at a great Expence, caused to be engraven for the Illustration of his *Microscopical Observations*, and which are, perhaps, the most valuable Part of the whole Work: for his Descriptive Accounts can, without the *Prints*, neither be instructive nor entertaining; but any tolerable Explanations may, with them, make a pretty good Amends for the Want of the MICROGRAPHIA.

To render them thus useful is the Design of this Undertaking; of which, as some little Account may reasonably be expected, it shall be given in as few Words as possible.

'Tis now seventy-nine Years since the MICROGRAPHIA was published; notwithstanding which, the *Copper-Plates* belonging to it were lately met with, well-preserved, and excepting a little Rust, which was easily cleared away, in as good Condition almost as ever: no more than one Impression, and that probably of no great Number, having been taken from them. Seven indeed were wanting to make up the whole Set compleat; but those are now supplied by exact Copies little or nothing inferior to the Originals.

As these were some of the first *Drawings* of Objects examined by the *Microscope*, so likewise are they, without Comparison, some of the best that were ever taken in so great a Number: here being no less than *Thirty-three Plates*, which contain a delightful Variety of Subjects, largely magnified, and curiously engraved

At the Time Dr. HOOKE published this Work, a verbose and diffused Way of Writing was in fashion, which seems to us at present tedious and distasteful, the Doctrine of equivocal Generation, or a spontaneous Production of many Species of minute Living-Creatures, as well as Vegetables, without any other Parents than Accident and Putrifaction, prevailed likewise almost universally, and had done so for Ages, however absurd it now appears to us: For which Reasons it has not been judged convenient to reprint the MICROGRAPHIA, but to give rather some short and plain Descriptions of its *Pictures*, without meddling at all with its *Opinions* or *Hypotheses*.

The

THE PREFACE.

The following Sheets are therefore drawn up as an Explanation of thefe *Copper-Plates*, and 'tis hoped they may even make them better underftood than they could be by the *Doctor's* own Accounts; which muft be acknowledged (with all due Regard to the Memory of fo great a Man) to be frequently tedious and obfcure, as well as fo unmethodical, that to feveral *Figures* no Defcriptions can poffibly be found, but by turning over the whole Book, there being no Direction at all to guide us to them.

It was neceffary to form thefe *Explanations* from the Work itfelf whereto the *Plates* belonged, but the Difpofition, Stile, and Manner, will be found entirely new: Whatever properly concerns the fame Subject being here brought together, from the different Places where fcattered and intermixed throughout the MICROGRAPHIA, and expreffed with the utmoft Brevity and Plainnefs of Language

This renders the prefent *Volume* fo fmall: though it really contains the whole Senfe of all that is neceffary fully to underftand the following *Plates*. And nearly one half, even of this Little, confifts of new *Difcoveries* or *Obfervations*, made fince the DOCTOR's Time, on the feveral Subjects which the *Figures* reprefent: whereby a great Variety of *Natural Hiftory* is conveyed to the READER's Hands, in a narrow Compafs and at a fmall Expence.——The *Plates* themfelves will be found alfo more inftructive, by engraving over every *Figure* an Account of what it is, and of the Page where we may look for the Defcription of it.

Little more is requifite than to inform the Reader, that the *Microfcope* Dr. HOOKE ufed was of the *Double-Kind*; but much more cumberfome, and lefs convenient, both as to its Structure and Apparatus than what our *Opticians* make at prefent. For this Inftrument (that new Sort particularly which has very lately been conftructed on an improved Plan) is brought now to fuch a Degree of Perfection, that no Obferver need be apprehenfive he fhall be unable to difcover, and that too very eafily, any of the minuteft Parts of Objects which the *Doctor* could difcern with the *Microfcope* he employed.

The *Doctor* fometimes mentions the comparative Size of Objects when magnified by his Glaffes; and therefore, as the *Curious* may very naturally enquire by what means he could compute their Bignefs, it feems proper to acquaint them with the Method whereby he took their Meafure.——Having (he tells us) rectified the *Microfcope*, to fee the defired Object through it very diftinctly; at the fame time that he look'd upon the Object through the Glafs with one Eye, he looked upon other Objects at the fame Diftance with his other bare Eye: by which means he was able, by the Help of a Ruler divided into Inches and fmall Parts, and laid on the Pedeftal of the *Microfcope*, to caft, as it were, the magnified Appearance of the Object upon the Ruler, and thereby exactly to meafure the Diameter it appears of through the Glafs; which being compared with the Diameter it appears of to the naked Eye, will eafily afford the Quantity of its being magnified.

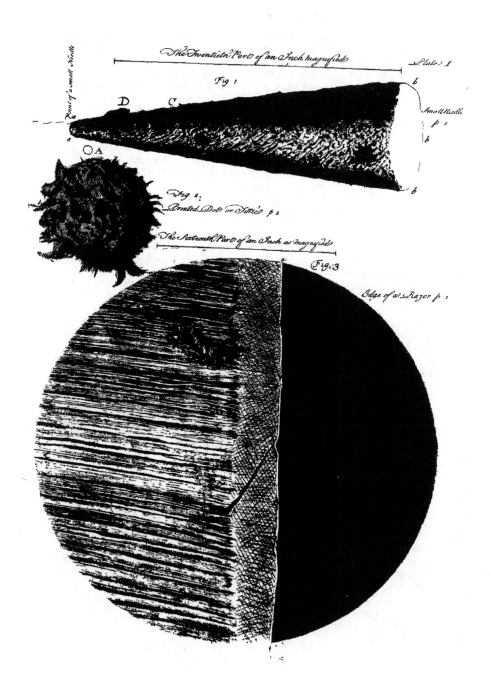

The Twentieth Part of an Inch magnified

Plate I

Fig 1

Point of a small Needle

D   C

b

Small Needle p. 1

b

O A

b

Fig 2:
Printed Dot or Tittle p. 1

The Sixteenth Part of an Inch as magnified

Fig: 3

Edge of a Razor p. 1

Micrographia Reſtaurata, &c.

An EXPLANATION of the FIRST PLATE.

FIG. I.

The Point of a ſmall ſharp Needle.

The Point of a Needle

DR HOOKE begins his Microſcopical Experiments with obſerving, that it is as requiſite, in the Study of Nature, to make ourſelves acquainted with the moſt ſimple and uncompounded Bodies, before we venture to examine thoſe of a more complicated kind, as it is to learn how to make our Letters before we pretend to write And, in conſequence of this Obſervation, the firſt Object he lays before us, comes the neareſt to a phyſical Point of any artificial thing we are acquainted with, I mean the Point of a ſmall Needle, made ſo ſharp that the naked Eye is unable to diſtinguiſh any of its Parts. This, notwithſtanding, appeared before his Microſcope as in the Figure at *a a*, where the very Top of the Needle is ſhewn above a Quarter of an Inch broad, not round or flat, but irregular and uneven.

The whole Piece we have here the Picture of, (according to the Scale given with it) is little more than the twentieth Part of an Inch in Length, and appeared to the naked Eye exquiſitely ſmooth and poliſhed, but, as ſeen by the Microſcope, what a Multitude of Holes and Scratches are diſcovered to us? How uneven and rough the Surface! how void of Beauty! and how plain a Proof of the Deficiency and Bunglingneſs of Art, whoſe Productions when moſt laboured, if examined with Organs more acute than thoſe by which they were framed, loſe all that fancied Perfection our Blindneſs made us think they had! Whereas, in the Works of Nature, the farther, the deeper our Diſcoveries reach, the more ſenſible we become of their Beauties and Excellencies

But to return to the Object now before us, A, B, C, repreſent large Hollows and Roughneſſes, like thoſe eaten into an Iron-Bar by Ruſt and Length of Time. D is ſome ſmall adventitious Body ſticking thereto by Accident.

b b b. ſhew the End where this ſmall Piece of Needle was broken off, in order to take the better View of it.

As ſharp as a Needle is a common Phraſe, whereby we intend to expreſs the moſt exquiſite Degree of Sharpneſs, and, indeed, a Needle has the moſt acute Point Art is capable of making, however rude and clumſy it appears when thus examined. But the Microſcope can afford us numberleſs Inſtances, in the Hairs, Briſtles, and Claws of Inſects, and alſo in the Thorns, Hooks, and Hairs of Vegetables, of viſible Points many Thouſands of times ſharper, with a Form and Poliſh that proclaim the Omnipotence of their Maker

PLATE I. FIG. 2.

A Printed Dot or Tittle.

A Dot or Tittle

WE have now before us the Repreſentation of a printed *Tittle*, or *Period Point*, as it appeared before the Microſcope To the naked Eye it was no larger than the Dot in the Middle of the Circle A, perfectly black and round, but through the Magnifier it ſeemed grey, and quite irregular, like a great Splatch of *London* Dirt, about three Inches over.

This rugged and deformed Appearance is owing to the uneven Surface of the Paper, (which looks at beſt no ſmoother than a very coarſe Piece of Shag-Cloth) added to the

Inc-

Irregularity of the Type, the rough dawbing of the Printing-Ink thereon, and the Variation made by the different Lights and Shadows. Nor is a Point made with a Pen, or by a Copper-Plate, at all lefs ill-fhapen and ugly; nor can the fineft Writing in the World ftand the Teft of this Inftrument, but will appear before it like the bungling Scrawls of a School-Boy, made with Charcoal on a whited Wall

PLATE I. FIG. 3.

The Edge of a Razor.

The Edge of a Razor

THIS *Figure* reprefents the Edge (about half a Quarter of an Inch long) of a very fharp Razor well fet upon a good Hone, and fo placed between the Object-Glafs and the Light, that there appeared a Reflection from the very Edge, which is fhewn by the white Line *a, b, c, d, e, f*

When we fpeak of any thing as extremely keen, we ufually compare it to the Edge of a Razor, but we find, when examined thus, how far from Sharpnefs even a Razor's Edge appears· That it feems a rough Surface, of an unequal Breadth from fide to fide, but fcarce any where narrower than the Back of a pretty thick Knife: That it is neither fmooth, even, nor regular, for it is fomewhat fharper than elfewhere at *d*, indented about *b*, broader and thicker about *c*, unequal and rugged about *e*, and moft even between *a, b,* and *e, f,* though very far in any Place from being really ftraight

The Side immediately below the Edge, and what the naked Eye accounts a Part of it, *g, h, y, k,* had nothing of that Polifh one would imagine Bodies fo fmooth as a Hone and Oil fhould give it, but was full of innumerable Scratches croffing one another, with Lines here and there, more rugged and deep than the reft, fuch as *g, h, y, k, o,* occafioned probably by fome fmall Duft falling on the Hone, or fome more flinty Part of the Hone itfelf.

The other Part of the Razor *L L*, which had been polifhed on a Grind-ftone, appeared like a plowed Field, full of Ridges and Furrows

The irregular dark Spot *m, n,* feemed to be a little Speck of Ruft, corrofive Juices generally working in fuch a manner.

This Examination proves, how rough and unfeemly (had we microfcopic Eyes) thofe Things would appear, which now the Dulnefs of our Sight makes us think extremely neat and curious. And, indeed, it feems impoffible by Art to give a perfect Smoothnefs to any hard and brittle Body, for *Putty,* or any other foft Powder, employed to polifh fuch Body, muft neceffarily confift of little hard rough Particles, each whereof cutting its Way, muft confequently leave fome kind of Furrow behind it In fhort, this Edge of a Razor, had it been really as the Microfcope fhews it, would fcarce have ferved to chop Wood, inftead of fhaving a Man's Beard

N B The black Part of this *Figure* is only defigned to make the reft more vifible. The Scale is intended to meafure the *Figure* by.

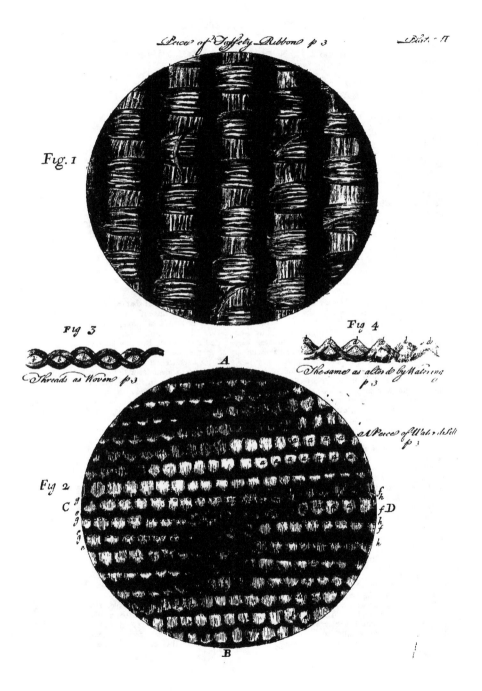

Peece of Taffety Ribbon p 3

Plat. II

Fig. 1

Fig 3

Threads as Woven p 3

Fig 4

The same as alterd by Watering p 3

A

A Peece of Waterd Silk p 3

Fig 2

C

D

B

An EXPLANATION of the SECOND PLATE.

FIG. 1.

A Piece of fine wheal'd Taffety Ribbon.

THIS Object was Sixpenny broad Ribbon, whose Substance viewed through the larger A Piece of Magnifying-Glass, appeared like Matting for Doors, or such Basket-Work as they Ribbon make in some Parts of *England*, for Bee-Hives, &c. with Straws a little wreathed or twisted. for every Filament of the Silk (several whereof go to the forming one Thread) seemed about the Size of a common Straw, as the little irregular Pieces *a b, c d, e f,* shew.

Each Inch of this Ribbon appeared no less than twelve Foot square, and an Inch and a half in Thickness. The *Warp* or *cross Threads* seemed like Ropes of an Inch Diameter, but the *longitudinal Threads* or *Woof* had scarce half that Thickness. If the Silk be white, it resembles Bundles or Wreaths of very clear and transparent Cylinders: if colour'd, each Cylinder, in some Place or other, affords as lively a Reflection as if it were made of Glass; insomuch that a Piece of red Ribbon exhibited as bright a Lustre as if coming from many Rubies. But such vivid Reflections are not found in hairy Stuffs or Linens.

PLATE II.   FIG. 2, 3, 4.

A Piece of Watered Silk.

THIS Figure represents a Piece of Watered Silk, as seen through a Glass that magnified A Piece of but little. A B signifies the long Way, C D the broad Way thereof Watered Silk

This Silk appeared to the naked Eye, waved, undulated, or grain'd all over, with so curious though irregular a Variety of brighter and darker Parts as much increased its Beauty. So well known a Case seems to need very little Explication · But few perhaps have considered, that those which in one Position appear to the Light the darker Parts of the Wave, in another appear the lighter, and *vice versâ* ; by which means the Undulations are continually shifting, as the Position of the Parts to the incident Beams of Light is varied. The Microscope discovers this Effect to proceed entirely from the Variety of the Reflections of Light, which the different Shape of the Particles, or the little Protuberances of the Threads composing the Surface occasion. Those Parts of the Waves that appear the brighter, throwing towards the Eye a Multitude of small Reflections, while the darker afford scarce any.

Thus, in the present Figure, the brighter Parts of the Surface, denoted by *a, a, a, a, a,* &c. consist of an Abundance of large and strong Reflections, the Surfaces of those Threads that run the long Way, being, by the mechanical Process of *Watering*, plaited or angled in another Form than they were by *Weaving*, for, by weaving, they are only turned circularly over and under the warping Threads, but by the Watering they are bent with an Angle or Elbow.

What is meant hereby will better be explained by the third and fourth Figures ; the Fig 3 former of which, *Fig.* 3. *a, a, a, a, a,* shews the Manner how the long Threads in Weaving are turned over and under the cross Threads, the Ends whereof are represented *b, b, b, b.*

Fig 4 shews how the same Threads are by the Watering bent and alter'd into An-Fig 4 gles or Elbows of all imaginable Variety ; whereby, instead of reflecting the Light from one Point only of the round Surface, as about *c, c, c :* they now, when watered, reflect its Beams from more than half the Surface, as, *d e, d e, d e.* These Reflections are also varied, as the particular Parts thereof are variously bent.

Dr. HOOKE, to make this fully understood, subjoins the Method of watering Silks or Stuffs ; the Substance of which, as being curious in itself, and necessary for the Explanation of the Figures, we shall give with all the Brevity possible.

The Piece to be watered must be doubled its whole Length, with the right Side inwards, exactly through the Middle, placing the two Selvedges just upon one another, and so disposing the Wheal or Rib in the doubling of it, that the Wheal of one Side may lie as near as can be parallel with that on the other, for the nearer they come to that Position, the greater appears the Watering, and the more obliquely they lie to each other, the Waves become the smaller.

The

The Way of folding it for a large Wheal is thus:---They take a Pin, and beginning at one Side of the Piece in any Wheal, direct it towards the End of the fame Wheal on the other Side, and then place the two oppofite Ends of the Wheal as near as they can together, and fo double or fold the whole Piece, repeating this Enquiry with a Pin at every Yard or two. This done, they fprinkle it with Water, and fold it the long Way, placing a Piece of Pafteboard between every Fold, whereby the Wheals on the wrong Side are flatten'd, and thofe on the Right become the more protuberant, and the angular Bendings of the Wheals are the more remarkable.

Being folded thus, they prefs it, between Pafteboards, violently, in a Hot-Prefs, and let it remain there till ftiff and dry, which makes the Wheals of the contiguous Sides leave Impreffions mutually on one another, as *Fig.* 2. demonftrates: where it is evident that the Wheal of the Piece A B C D runs parallel between the pricked Lines *ef, ef, ef*; and Impreffions being left upon thefe Wheals by thofe that were preft upon them, (which lay not exactly parallel to, but a little athwart them, as the Lines *o o o o o o o, g b, g b, g b,* fhew) they are fo varioufly and irregularly creafed, and their Threads fo fet to each other, by being put into that Shape when wet, and kept fo till dry, that the Mouldings will remain almoft as long as the Silk itfelf.

Hence any one that confiders the Figure attentively, will be fenfible, why the Parts of the Wheal *a a a a a a* appear bright, the Parts *b b b b b b* dark or fhadowed, and fome fuch as *d d d d d* partly light and partly dark. The Variety of which Reflections and Shadows are the only Caufe of the Appearance we call *Watering* in Silks or Stuffs.

Fine Lawn.

Fine Lawn

A Piece of the fineft Lawn, whofe Threads are fcarce difcernable by the naked Eye, appears through the Microfcope coarfer than any Hop-Sack; its Threads feeming not unlike, either in Shape or Size, the larger Kind of *Rope-Yarn,* wherewith they ufually make Cables: And its Tranfparency is plainly feen to arife from a Multitude of fquare Holes, left between the Threads, which give it the Refemblance of a Lattice-Window, only here the croffing Parts are round and not flat. Thefe Threads, however, though as fmall as in the fineft Silks, have nothing of their gloffy, pleafant and lively Reflections.

A Drawing of this is given, *Plate* XI. *Fig* 3.

Our Author proceeds no farther in examining the Productions of human Art, Things only defigned to be viewed by our naked Eyes, and wherein little is difcoverable but Rudenefs and Deformity, but applies his Microfcope to behold the minute Works of Nature, which though far removed beyond the Reach of our Sight, are fo exquifitely curious, that the more our Glaffes magnify the more Excellencies appear therein, the more we learn the Weaknefs of ourfelves, and the Omnipotency and infinite Perfections of the Great Creator.

Plate III

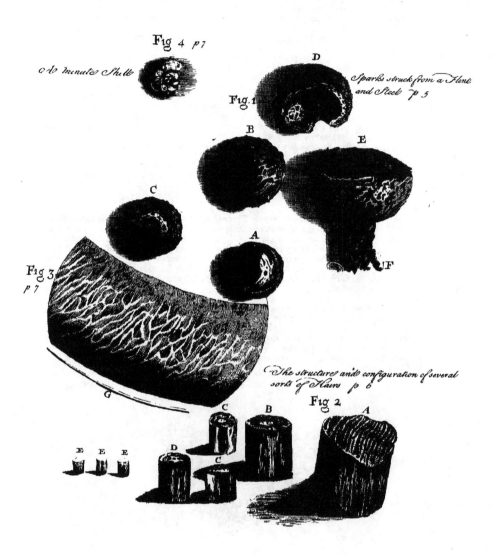

Fig 4 *p 7*

A minute Shell

D

Fig. 1

Sparks struck from a Flint and Steel p 5

B

E

C

A

Fig 3 *p 7*

F

G

The structures and configuration of several sorts of Hairs p 6

Fig 2

C B A

E E E D C

An EXPLANATION of the THIRD PLATE.

FIG. 1.

The Sparks of Fire ſtruck from a Flint and Steel.

IN the common Way of ſtriking Fire with a Flint and Steel, fiery Sparks fly out at *Globules of* every Blow ; which Sparks are nothing more than ſmall Pieces of the Flint or Steel, *Steel* (but uſually of the Steel) broken off by the Violence of the Stroke, and either melted inſtantaneouſly into Steel Globules, or made at leaſt red-hot, and thereby capable of kindling Tinder or Touch-wood. The Heat is likewiſe ſo intenſe ſometimes as even to vitrify the broken Particles.

As a Proof of this, Dr. HOOKE ſtruck Fire over a Sheet of very white Paper, and obſerving diligently where the Sparks ſeemed to vaniſh, he diſcovered there certain very ſmall, black, but glittering and moveable Specks, which, when examined with his Microſcope, appeared to be little round Globules, ſome whereof did, from their Surface, yield a very bright and ſtrong Reflection on that Side next the Light, and reſembled Iron-Balls. One of which, whoſe Surface was pretty regular, is ſhewn by the Letter A.

He perceived in this the reflected Image of the Window, and alſo of a Stick, which he moved up and down between the Light and it

He found others almoſt regularly round, as to the Bulk of the Ball, but with rough unpoliſhed Surfaces, which rendered the Reflection from them much more confuſed and faint. Such are repreſented by the Letters B, C, D, E.

Some were cracked or cleft, as C ; others broken and quite hollow, as D ; which ſeemed like half the hollow Shell of a Granado, broken irregularly in Pieces. There were other different Shapes, but that in particular, marked with the Letter E, was a larger Spark of Fire than ordinary. It went out on one Side the Flint employed in ſtriking it, and adhered thereto by the Root F. On the Top of its Stem was faſtned half an hollow Ball, with the Mouth of it opening upwards, ſo that it appeared ſomewhat like a Funnel, or a Rummer-Glaſs without a Foot.

The melting of the Particles of Steel, inſtantaneouſly, upon the Colliſion, is very wonderful, and comes up nearly to the Effects of Lightning. Indeed there ſeems to be in Iron or Steel a ſulphureous combuſtible Matter very eaſily put in Action, for either hammering, filing, or rubbing it with Violence, will preſently make it ſo hot as to be able to burn one's Finger And if the Filings of Iron are only let drop through the Flame of a Candle, (placing a Sheet of white Paper underneath, to catch them for Examination) many of them will be found melted even by that ſudden Tranſit, and appear remarkably ſhining to the naked Eye, and if we view them farther by the Microſcope, we ſhall ſoon be ſatisfied they are exactly ſuch round Globules as are formed by ſtriking Fire with a Flint and Steel.

As obtaining ſuch minute Globules as theſe, of Lead or Tin, and that even in Quan- *Globules of* tity, eaſily and quickly, may be deſirable by ſome, we ſhall here ſubjoin the Way of *Lead or Tin* forming them, which Dr HOOKE ſays a learned Phyſician taught him.

Reduce the Metal you would ſhape thus, into exceedingly fine Filings : for the ſmaller your Filings are, the ſmaller will be your Globules. Strew ſome fine and well-dried Powder of Quick-Lime at the Bottom of a Crucible, on which ſcatter ſome of your Filings very thinly, then ſtrew on more Powder, on that again more Filings, and ſo alternately, Stratum ſuper Stratum, till you have filled your Crucible, in ſuch a manner, that, as near as may be, no two Filings may touch each other. Place the Crucible in a gradual Fire, and increaſe the Heat by Degrees, till it be ſufficient to make all the Filings mix'd with the Quick-Lime melt, and no more. For if the Fire be too hot, many of the Filings will join and run together : But if the Heat be duly proportioned, upon waſhing the Lime-Duſt in Water, all thoſe ſmall Filings of the Metal will ſubſide to the Bottom, in a moſt curious Powder, conſiſting of Balls or Globules exactly round, which, if very fine, is excellent for Hour Glaſſes.

One may, at any time, procure immediately minute Globules of Lead, by only *Globules of* kindling a red Wafer, ſuch as Letters are ſealed with, at a Candle, for as it burns (and *Lead* it will not go out till it be wholly conſumed) the red Lead employed in the Colouring, melts, and falls down, in regular minute Globules, which, if a Sheet of clean *wh te*

C

white Paper be placed underneath, may be catched in greater Abundance than can be imagined without Trial.

PLATE III.   FIG. 2.

The Structure and Configuration of several Sorts of Hairs.

Bristles of an Hog

THE Bristles of an Hog were found of a Substance hard, transparent, and horny, without the least Appearance of Pores or Holes, as was tried by cutting them transversely with a sharp Razor, and then examining their cut Ends by a Microscope. This shewed many wavy Figures thereon, occasioned by the Sawing of the Razor to and fro, as we may see at the End of the Body A   But notwithstanding Light was cast upon them all the various Ways that could be thought on, to make the Pores visible, none at all could be discovered.

They were neither perfectly round, nor sharp-edged, but prismatical, with divers Sides and round Angles, *Vid.* A.   Bending them in any Part takes away the Transparency where the Bending is, makes them look white, and flaws them in that Place.

Whiskers of a Cat

B represents the Whisker of a Cat cut the cross Way, in the Middle whereof a large Pith appeared like the Pith of Elder, whose Texture was so compact that no Pores could be discovered in it, for tho' in one Position to the Light there seemed an Appearance of Pores, that Position being alter'd, the Light was manifestly reflected from them.   Which may serve as a Caution never to conclude too rashly on what we view through Microscopes, or declare our Opinion till we have examined Things in every Light and Position, and by all the Contrivances in our Power.

Horse Hair

C C, and D, are Pieces of the long Hairs of Horses, which appear cylindrical and somewhat pithy

Human Hair

E E E represent three Sections of the Hairs of a Man's Head, which were found generally almost round, though sometimes a little prismatical.   The Part next the Top was bigger than that nearer the Root.   They were throughout transparent, though not very clear, nor every where of the same Colour, being near the Root like black transparent Horn, but near the Top-Extremity like Horn that is clear and brown.   Their Roots were pretty smooth, tapering upwards like a small Parsnep, nor could any Filaments, or other Vessels, like Fibres from the Roots of Plants, be found.

The Top when split, which is common in long Hair, appeared like the End of a Stick shivered with Beating, with sometimes half a Score Splinters or Divisions.

Our Author says, that as far as he could find, Human Hairs are all solid cylindrical Bodies, not pervious like a Cane or Bulrush, but without any Pith or Distinction of Rind, and imagines those who assert them to be hollow, have not inspected them with sufficient Care.

Dr Power *, on the contrary, makes no doubt that every one of our Hairs is hollow, which, though our Glasses cannot demonstrate, by reason of their Transparency, is palpably evinced by that Disease in *Poland* called the *Plica*, where Blood drops from the Ends of the Hairs of the Head, and likewise issues out wherever they are cut, which, he thinks, infallibly proves the tubulous Cavity of them.   But to this Dr. Hooke answers, that the Microscope gives no Encouragement to believe our Hairs are hollow, and that perhaps the very Essence of the Distemper called the *Plica Polonica*, may be their growing hollow, and of an unnatural Constitution

Malpighi asserts the Hairs of Animals to be tubular, that is, composed of a Number of extremely minute Tubes or Pipes, which he concludes from his Examination of a Horse's Main and Tail, and the Bristles of a Boar.   These Tubes were most distinguishable near the End of the Hairs where they appeared more open ·   And he sometimes could reckon above twenty of them.   He perceived these Tubes very plainly in the Hedge-Hog's Prickles, (which are of the Nature of Hairs) together with elegant medullary Valves and Cells

Mr. Leeuwenhoek tells us, that an human Hair, cut transversely, shews a Variety of Vessels in regular Figures.

* *Power's* Exper p 56

1   PLATE

PLATE III. FIG. 3.

Hair of an Indian Deer.

F Exhibits the Middle Part of the Hair of an *Indian* Deer, and G the Top or Extremity of the fame Hair, both magnified by the fame Glafs, whereby is fhewn how extremely tapering thefe Hairs are formed, which indeed was obfervable by the naked Eye; for though in the Middle it was thicker than an Hog's Briftle, it was flenderer at the End than the Hair of any other Animal. The whole Belly of it was two or three Inches long, and appeared to the Eye like a Thread of coarfe Canvas that has newly been unravelled, being all bent or waved to and fro, in the Manner of fuch a Thread. But feen through the Microfcope, it feemed all perforated from Side to Side, and fpongy; and refembled a fmall Kind of fpongy Coral, found frequently on the Coafts of *England*. When cut tranfverfely, no Pores could be difcerned running the long Way of the Hair.

The Hairs of different Animals are curious Objects for the Microfcope. In fome tranfverfe, in other fpinal Lines, fomewhat of a darker Colour, run from Bottom to Top, in a very pretty Manner. A Moufe's Hairs are of this Sort. They appear as it were in Joints like the Back-Bone, are not fmooth, but jagged on the Sides, and terminate in the fharpeft Point imaginable. Hairs taken from a Moufe's Belly are leaft opake, and fitteft for Examination *.

Hairs taken from the Head, the Eye-Brows, the Noftrils, the Beard, the Hand, and other Parts of the Body, appear unlike, as well in the Roots as in the Hair themfelves, and vary as Plants do of the fame *Genus*, but of different *Species*. They all become lengthened by Propulfion, and are thicker towards the Middle than at either End.

PLATE III. FIG. 4.

A pretty minute Shell found amongft Sand.

T HIS Shell appeared to the naked Eye like a white Spot, no bigger than the Point of a Pin, but when viewed by the Microfcope, it was found in every Particular to refemble the flat fpiral Shell of a Water Snail, and had twelve Wreathings, *a, b, c, d, e,* &c. all diminifhing gradually towards the Middle or Center, where there was a very fmall, round, white Spot. 'Twas not eafy to difcover whether it was hollow or not, but it rather feemed to be filled with fomewhat, and probably might be petrified, as larger Shells are often.

The Object under Obfervation informs us of another *Genus*, where the Almighty Hand of the Maker is amazingly exemplified in the Minutenefs and Elegance of the Work: For we find hereby that the fame Power which contrived fuch minute Infects as Mites, fuch minute Fifhes as the Eels in Vinegar, and fuch minute Vegetables as Mofs and Mouldinefs, has likewife formed a Tribe of fuch minute Shells as this before us, the Beauty of which could never have been difcovered without the Microfcope's Affiftance. It was found, accidentally, amongft fome White-fand that was looked at with no other Defign than to try the Goodnefs of fome Glaffes: But many valuable Difcoveries have been owing to lucky Accident.

* Microfcope made eafy, p 245.

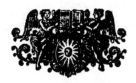

An EXPLANATION of the FOURTH PLATE.

FIG. I.

Some curious Forms of fmall Diamonds, or fhining Sparks in Flints.

Diamonds in
Flints

BReaking a Flint-Stone by Accident, a Cavity was found therein, all crufted over with a pretty candy'd Subftance, A A, &c. fome Parts of which, fuch as B B B B, on turning them to the Light, reflected its Rays in a very glittering and lively Manner And bringing it to the Microfcope, the whole Surface of the Cavity appeared befet with a Multitude of little chryftalline or Diamond-like Bodies, curioufly fhaped and polifhed, as the Drawing reprefents them.

The vivid Repercuffions of Light were, on Examination, obferved to be reflected partly from the plain external Surfaces of thefe regularly figured Bodies, and partly from within the pellucid Bodies themfelves, that is, from fome Surfaces thereof oppofite to thofe Surfaces which were next the Eye.

But thefe Sparks being fo fmall, that no certain Experiments could eafily be made with them, Dr. HOOKE procured feveral of the fhining Stones or Chryftals found in great Quantities in *Cornwall*, and therefore called moft commonly *Cornifh* Diamonds; which growing in the hollow Cavities of Rocks, much after the fame manner as thefe did in the Flint, and having regularly-fhaped Surfaces nearly of the fame Form with theirs, he imagined might afford fome convenient Help towards afcertaining the Properties of fuch Kinds of Bodies.

By thefe he found, that the brighteft Reflections of Light proceeded from within the pellucid Body , that is, the Rays admitted through the pellucid Subftance, in their getting out on the oppofite Side, were very vividly reflected by the contiguous and ftrong reflecting Surface of the Air, fo that more Rays were reflected to the Eye by this Surface, (though the Ray in entering and getting out of the Chryftal had fuffered a double Refraction) than there were from the outward Surface of the Glafs, where it had fuffered no Refraction at all.

Sands

It is proper here to take notice, that our Author mentions his Examination of feveral Sorts of Sands with his Microfcope, amongft which he found divers moft curioufly fhaped, as thefe in the Flint were, and which, he therefore fuppofes, not made by the Comminution of larger chryftalline Bodies, but formed by the Concretion or Coagulation of Water, or fome other Fluid.

Sand, however, generally feems nothing elfe but exceeding fmall Pebbles, or fome fmall Pieces of bigger Stones, angled for the moft part irregularly, without any certain Shape, and having its little Grains frequently flawed and broken.

There are many Sorts of Sands, (as many perhaps as there are of Stones) which differ from one another both in Colour, Figure, and Size. And as amongft Stones fome are called precious for their Excellency, fo alfo amongft Sands, there are fome that deferve the fame Epithet for their Beauty. The Grains of *Sea-Sands* are very large, and afford great Variety of all Shapes and Colour-, both opake and tranfparent. *River-Sands* are fmaller-grained, of different Colours and Forms, and the *Inland* or *Pit-Sands*, vary alfo exceedingly, being fome white, fome brown, fome yellow, &c.

The *white*, or *Writing-Sand*, appears through the Microfcope like tranfparent Pieces of *Allum*, *Sal-Gem*, or *Chryftal*, but moft commonly irregular. The *coarfer Sands* are ufually more opake, but even amongft them many Grains may be found both clear and beautiful. Some Kinds of *black Sand* are brought from the *Eaft-Indies*, and likewife from *Virginia* and other Parts of *America*, with polifhed fhining Surfaces, many of which will be attracted by the Load-ftone, and there are certain *reddifh Sands* (brought from abroad alfo) which prefent a delightful Sight to the Eye, not unlike a Jeweller's Box of Treafure, wherein you fee *Rubies* of a Rofe-Colour, others of a deeper Red, *Sapphires*, *Emeralds*, *Hyacinths*, *Topazes*, and in fhort, all Sorts of tranfparent Stones *.

* Spectacle de la Nat Dial XIX

Plate IV

Regularly Figured Chrystal or Diamonds in the Cavity of a Flint Stone

Fig. I

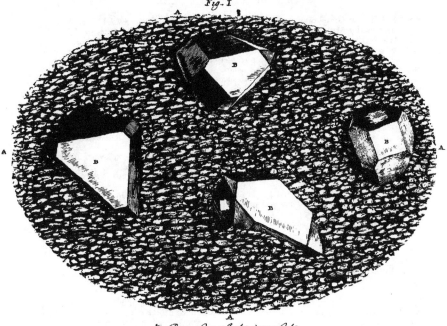

To Part of an Inch magnified

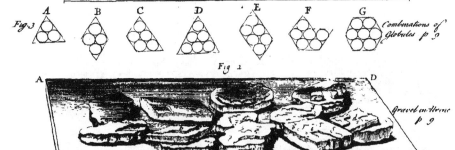

Fig 3

A   B   C   D   E   F   G   *Combinations of Globules p. 9*

Fig 2

A   D

Gravel in Verne p 9

B   C

Sr Part of an Inch magnified

Fig 4

 H    I   K    L   *More Combinations of Globules p. 9*

PLATE IV. FIG. 2.

The Forms of Gravel in Urine.

THE Sand or Gravel of Urine seems to be a tartareous Substance, generated of saline Gravel in and earthy Matter chrystalized together, sticking sometimes to the Sides of the Urine Chamber-Pot, but more frequently sinking to the Bottom, and there appearing in the Form of coarse Sand, the Grains whereof, seen through the Microscope, resemble a Company of small Bodies, partly transparent, and partly opake, some white, some yellow, some red, and others of more brown and dusky Colours.

In Shape they are mostly flat, after the Manner of Slates, or such-like plated Stones, and seem composed of several very thin *Lamellæ*, like *Muscovy Glass* or *English Spar*, the latter of which they appear nearly to resemble, having their Sides, as that has, form'd into Rhombs, or Rhomboids, and sometimes into Rectangles and Squares

The Figure under our Eye represents a Dozen of them, (as examined by the Microscope, lying on a Slip of Glass, A B C D, some whereof, as *a, b, c, d,* were more regular than the rest, and *e,* a small one, sticking upon another, was a perfect Rhomboid on the Top, and had four rectangular Sides.

Their Bigness is shewn by the Line E, which was the Measure of the Microscope, and a Scale of the thirty-second Part of an Inch magnified, by this Measure it is evident, that none of them exceeded in Breadth, the one hundred and twenty-eighth Part of an Inch

Oil of Vitriol, Spirit of Urine, and several *saline Menstrua,* dissolved them in a Minute or two without any Ebullition: *Water* and many other Liquors had no sudden Effect upon them Such Fluids as dissolve them, render them very white at first, not spoiling but rather rectifying their Figures, and making them more agreeable Objects for the Microscope.

PLATE IV.　FIG. 3, and 4.

A Variety of regular Forms resulting from various Combinations of Globules.

DR HOOKE imagines the Chrystalization of Salts, and all those regular Figures that Effects of a are so remarkably various and curious, and beautify such Multitudes of Bodies, arise Combination only from three or four different Positions of *globular Particles,* and those the most plain, of Globules obvious, and necessary Conjunctions of such *figured Particles* that can possibly happen So that, supposing such plain and obvious Causes concurring, the *coagulating Particles* must, as necessarily, compose a Body of such a determinate regular Figure, and no other, as a fluid Body encompassed with an heterogeneous Fluid must be rounded into a Globule or Sphere And he says, he has demonstrated, only by a Company of Bullets, and one or two other very simple Bodies, that merely almost by shaking them together, he could make them compose any regular Figure he had ever met with

For Example. If a Number of Bullets be put on an inclining Plane, so that they may run together, they will fall, naturally, into a *triangular Order,* composing all the Variety of Figures that can be imagined to be made out of *æquilateral Triangles,* such as all the Surfaces of *Alum,* upon Examination, will be found to be, for three Bullets lying on a Plane, as close as they can to one another, compose an *æquilateral-triangular* Form, as is shewn at A

If a Fourth be joined to them, as closely as it can, on either Side, the four together form a most regular *Rhombus,* consisting of two *æquilateral Triangles,* as B.

If a Fifth be joined to them on either Side, in as close a Position as can be, (which is a Circumstance always to be understood in these Experiments) it makes a *Trapezium,* or *four-sided Figure,* two of whose Angles are 120, and the other two 60 Degrees, as C

On the Addition of a Sixth, as before, it makes either an *æquilateral Triangle,* like D, or a *Rhomboid,* as E, or an *hexangular* Figure composed of two primary *Rhombes,* as F.

If we add a Seventh, it makes either an *æquilatero-hexagonal* Figure, as G, or some kind of *six-sided* Figure, like H, or I

And though never so many be placed together, they may be all ranged under some of these before mentioned Forms, with Angles either of sixty, or one hundred and twenty

D　　　　　　　　　　　　　　　Degrees,

Degrees, as the Letter K fhews, which is an *æqui-angular hexagonal* Figure compounded of twelve Globules : And in the fame Manner, 25, or 27, or 36, or 42, &c. may be combined

Nor does it hold only in *Superficies*, but alfo in *Solidity* , for 'tis beyond Difpute, that if a *fourth* Globule be laid on the *third* in this Texture, it compofes a regular *Tetrahedron*, which is a very ufual Figure amongft the Chryftals of *Alum* And, indeed, amongft the Variety of regular Shapes into which the fmooth Surfaces of *Alum* are obferved to be chryftalized, there is not one but may be imitated by a fuch-like Pofition of Globules

The *cubical* Forms of *Sea-Salt* and *Sal-Gem*, are alfo (our Author fuppofes) compofed of fuch a Pofition of *Globules*, as the Letter L fhews. *Vitriol, Salt-Petre, Chryftal, Hore-Froft*, &c have likewife, he fays, all their various Configurations from *Globules* differently combined

---

An EXPLANATION of the FIFTH PLATE.

This Plate exhibits feveral Kinds of Figures produced by Freezing, which are extremely curious and wonderful, and deferve the Attention of all diligent Obfervers of the Works of Nature.

PLATE V. FIG. 1.

One of the Six-branched Figures on the Surface of Urine, when it begins to freeze.

Urine frozen THESE Figures had ufually a Center, *a*, from whence the Branches extended them-felves And wherever a Center was, the Branchings from it, *a b, a c, a d, a e, a f, a g*, were never more nor lefs than fix, which all iffued very nearly from the fame Point or Center *a*, tho' fometimes not exactly ; and inclined to one another, at an Angle of about fixty Degrees, without any fenfible Variation , but as the whole fix Branches compofed a folid Angle, they muft neceffarily be fomething lefs

The Middle-Lines or Stems of thefe Branches, *a b, a c, a d, a e, a f, a g*, appeared fomewhat whiter, and a little higher than any of the intermediate Lines, feeming to rife above the Surface of the Urine: And the Center *a* was evidently the moft prominent of the whole, refembling the *Apex* of a folid Angle or Pyramid.

The lateral Branchings from the fix large Stems, fuch as *o p, m q*, &c. were each of them inclined to the Stems from which they iffued, at the fame Angle (of about fixty De-grees) as the faid large Stems were to one another ; the bigger Branches always rifing higher than the lefs, and the lefs higher than the leaft, and fo in proportionate Gradations.

Thefe Side-Shoots were each of them parallel to that great Branch next which it lay , and all the Shoots on one Side were parallel to each other, as well as to the great Branch next them. For Example· The lateral Shoots *p o, q r*, are parallel to one another, and are alfo at the fame time parallel to the large Branch *a b*.

Some of the Stems proceeded ftrait, and decreafed in Thicknefs towards the End, as *a g*. Others grew bigger and knotty towards the Middle ; and the Side-Shootings, as well as the main Stems, from Cylinders became a Sort of femi-circular Planes, in a moft admirable and curious Order, and exceedingly delicate and regular, as may be feen at *a b, a c, a d, a e, a f*: (Thefe circular Figures, in the lateral Shoots, were alfo ftill more remarkable at *b s*) But towards the End of fome of thefe Stems, they began again to diminifh and recover their former Branchings, as about *k* and *n*

Such lateral Branches as *q m*, had many collateral Shootings, (if we may call them fo) as *f, t*, moft whereof had fub-collateral ones, as *v, w*, which again had others lefs, and thofe leffer ones had ftill minuter Shootings iffuing from them.

The Branchings from the main Stems were not joined by any regular Line, nor did the Side of one lie over that of the other, but in the fmall collateral and fub-collateral Shoot-ings, one Branch lay over the Side of the next that approached to it, as the Feathers do in a Bird's Wing See the *Figures* 1, 2, 3, 4, 5, 6, 7, 8, 9, 10.

Many fuch-like Configurations were obferved, of different Sizes, from the Bignefs of a Two-pence, to three or four Foot long, of which feveral were pretty round, having all

their

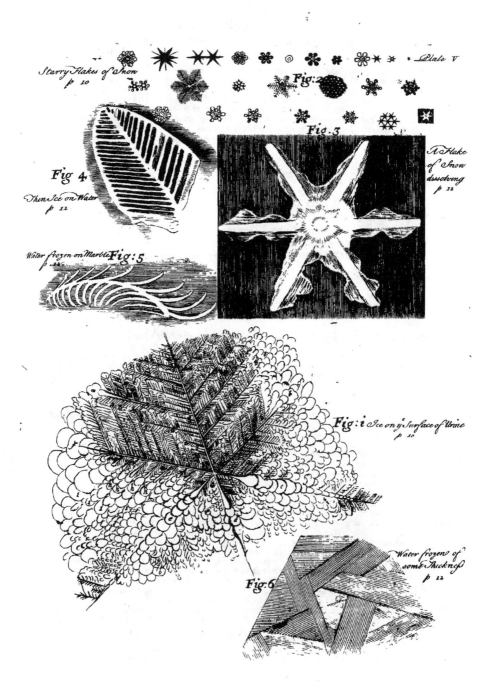

Plate V

Starry Flakes of Snow
p 10

Fig: 2.

Fig. 3

A Flake
of Snow
dissolving
p 12

Fig 4
Thin Ice on Water
p 12

Water frozen on Marble Fig: 5
p 12

Fig: 1 Ice on y.e Surface of Urine
p 10

Water frozen of
some Thickness
p 12

Fig: 6

their Branches near alike, but others were more extended towards one Side   None, how-ever, had any regular Pofition in refpect of one another, or of the Sides of the Veffel ; nor did any of them extend exactly every Way from the Center *a*

It is neceffary, in the Freezing of Urine for this Experiment, that its Superficies be not difturbed by Wind, or any other Way, and that it be not frozen too deep, for then the branched Appearance becomes loft.

If the Infide of a fmooth and clear Glafs be wetted with Urine, and expofed in a fharp Froft, it will be covered with very regular and curious Figures   But an artificial Freezing with Snow and Salt, produces not the natural Shootings in Urine, unlefs the Quantity in the Veffel be very fmall.

It is remarkable, that no urinous Tafte was perceived in feveral clear Pieces of fuch Ice, but they feemed as infipid as Water.

Somewhat like this Configuration of frozen Urine, tho' in fome Particulars much more curious, is obfervable in the *Regulus Martis Stellatus*, but whereas in this *Ice* the Stems and Branchings are all ftrait, in the *Regulus* they appear regularly bent or wreathed, in a very beautiful Manner. Lead and Arfenic, with fome other Mixtures, are alfo found to have their Surface, when fuffered to cool, with Branches not much unlike to thofe of Urine, but fmaller a great deal.

Dr Hooke takes occafion here to fhew the Refemblance of the Shootings before de- Like to Fern
fcribed, in *Urine*, to the Branchings in the Leaves of *Fern*, whofe Form, he fays, is the moft fimple and uncompounded of any Vegetable, except Mould or Mufhrooms : For the main Stem in *Fern* may be obferved to fend forth lateral Branches, from whence col-lateral ones arife, and from them again fub-collateral ones, after much the fame Order as the Branchings, Divifions and Subdivifions appear in the Figures of *frozen Urine*. He adds, that if both be well confidered, there feems not much greater Need of a *feminal Prin-ciple* to produce *Fern*, than for the Production of fuch Forms in *Urine*, or in the above-mentioned *Regulus Martis*, fince as much Beauty and Regularity appears in the one as in the other. And to this he fubjoins, that notwithftanding feveral have affirmed that *Fern* produces, and is propagated by Seed, he could never find any Part of it to be more feminal than another, tho' he had made very diligent Enquiry as to that Particular.

'Tis a little furprizing that our Author was not able, with his Microfcope, to difcover Seeds of Fern
the Seeds of this Plant, which produces them in the greateft Abundance on the Backs of almoft all its Leaves, in Seed-Veffels that appear to the naked Eye like a black or brown Scurf, but, when viewed by the Microfcope, refemble little circular Tubes di-vided into many Cells, containing Seeds extremely minute   When the Seed is ripe, the Veffels fly open with a Spring, and fquirt the Seeds out on every Side, in the Form of Duft. And if at that Seafon fome of the Leaves are put into a Paper-Cone, and that be held to the Ear, the Seed-Veffels may be heard to burft with a confiderable Noife   Some of thefe minute Veffels contain at leaft an hundred Seeds, invifible to the naked Eye

One may reafonably believe our Author never looked for them on the Backs of the Leaves, but finding neither Flowers nor Seeds in the fame manner as in other Plants, he concluded too haftily that it produced neither. Such Miftakes in great Men afford us ufeful Leffons of being very cautious in giving our Opinions, and never to determine be-fore we have examined fully.

PLATE V. FIG. 2.

The Forms of Falling Snow

THE Works of Nature are no lefs admirable for their Variety than their Beauty ! Flakes of
Even in fuch Things as appear the moft alike, a ftrict Examination will difcover Snow
to us Differences beyond all human Conception ! No two Grains of Sand are exactly fimilar ! Nay, the very Flakes of Snow afford an amazing Variety of Configuration, Beauty and Size, though not one in a Thoufand of thofe that fee them fall, either know or imagine any thing worth obferving in them

But Dr. Hooke tells us, that catching the falling Snow on a black Hat, or a Piece of black Cloth, he obferved the curious Figures of its Flakes with the utmoft Pleafure, and he prefents us, out of a great Variety, with the feveral beautiful Forms under our Eye at prefent

Every Flake confifts of fix principal Branches or Stems, all of equal Length, Shape, and Make, iffuing from a Center, and each of them inclining to the next on either Side it in an Angle of fixty Degrees.

Thefe

These Stems in the same Flake are commonly of the same Make exactly, but different in different Flakes, insomuch that, our Author says, he has observed above an hundred different Forms and Sizes of these Star-like Flakes fallen in a very little Time.

· The Branchings out from every Stem in the same Flake are so exactly alike, that only by observing the Configuration of any one Stem, one may know certainly the Figures of the other Side, the Branchings are likewise generally similar to those in frozen Urine before described

We have here before us six and twenty Representations of the Flakes of Snow, of different Shapes and Sizes, as they appear to the naked Eye   DES CARTES, Dr GREW, Mr. MORTON, Dr LANGWITH, and some others, have also given us many of their Star-like Forms, and Dr. STOCKE of *Zealand* lately communicated to the Royal Society several Figures observed and drawn by him, but differing very little from those of Dr. HOOKE *.

PLATE V.   FIG. 3.

A Flake of Snow magnified.

A Flake of
Snow mag-
nified

THE Flakes of Snow, examined by a Microscope, do not appear so perfectly regular and exact as might be expected, but, like Works of Human Art, the more they are magnified, the more misshapen and rude they seem; of which the Figure before us is a Specimen   This, however, is not owing to any Defect or Irregularity in their Formation, but to the unequal Thawing, or breaking of them as they fall   for I make no doubt, if it were possible to get a Sight of them through a Microscope as they are generated in the Clouds, and before their *Figures* are prejudiced by external Accidents, we should find them curiously beautiful, exact, and perfect.

PLATE V.   FIG. 4.

The Form of Ice on Water.

An Icicle

FAIR Water being exposed to the Cold in a capacious Vessel of Glass, after a little time, several broad, flat, and thin *Laminæ* or *Plates* of *Ice* were observed on the Surface, crossing the Water and each other very irregularly.   Most of them seemed to turn one of their Edges towards that Side of the Glass next it, and to grow as it were inwards towards the Middle of the Vessel.

Some of these *Laminæ* being taken out of the Water on the Blade of a Knife, were found to be figured after the Manner of *Herring-Bones*, or the Branches of *Fern*, having in the Middle one larger Stem, like the *Back-Bone*, and issuing out of it on either Side Multitudes of small Icicles, like the smaller Bones, or the smaller Branches in *Fern*.   Each of these Icicles was parallel to all the rest on the same Side, and all of them appeared to make an Angle with the Stem of about sixty Degrees.

PLATE V.   FIG. 5.

Ice on Marble.

Ice

A Little Water exposed to the Cold on a broad flat Marble, exhibited, when frozen, a very pretty Variety of Figures, some like Feathers, others of different Shapes, and many in the Appearance of the Picture here referred to

PLATE V.   FIG. 6.

Ice of another Configuration.

Ice

FLAKES of Ice frozen on the Top of Water to any considerable Thickness, were found, on Examination, to have both their Upper and Under-Sides curiously quill'd, furrow'd, or grained, which the Sun shining thereon shewed to be, as in the Drawing, several strait Ends of parallel Plates, of divers Lengths and Angles to one another, without any certain Order.

* Some of these Figures are printed in *Phil. Transf.* Numb. 464.

I

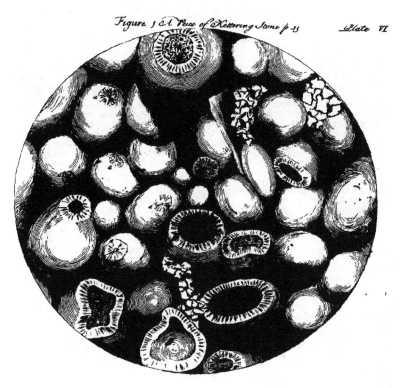

Figure 1 A Piece of Kettering Stone p 23   Plate VI

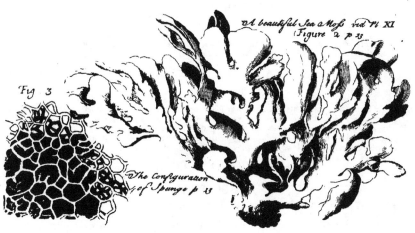

A beautiful Sea Moss vid Pl XI
(Figure 2 p 23

Fig 3

The Configuration
of Spunge p 23

An EXPLANATION of the SIXTH PLATE.

FIG. 1.

A Piece of Kettering-Stone.

THIS Stone, which has a very extraordinary Grain, much different from all other Kinds of Stone, is dug from a Quarry at *Kettering* in *Northamptonshire*. It appeared through the Microscope made up of numberless little Pebbles, whose Figure was nearly globular, though they were not all exactly of the same Shape or Bigness, some exceeding others three or four times in Diameter. They seemed, to the naked Eye, like the Ovary or Hard-Row of an Herring, or some smaller Fish; but the little Grains were neither so large nor so uniform. Their Variation in Shape from perfect Roundness looked as if occasioned entirely by the Pressure of some of the Balls against others, whereby the Sides where the Pressure took place, became a little depressed inwards, and the other Parts became protruded proportionably outwards, beyond the Limits of a Globe, in the same manner as it would happen, if an Heap of exactly round Balls of soft Clay were piled upon one another.

These Grains were so firmly united together where they touch each other, that they seldom could be parted without breaking an Hole in one or both, which Fractures are shewn by *a, a, a, b, c c,* &c.

In several, where the Pressure had been but light, no more was broken than the outward Crust or Shell of the Stone, which appeared of a white Colour, dash'd a little with a brownish yellow, and very thin like the Shell of an Egg. Nay, some of those Grains were found perfectly to resemble Eggs both in Colour and Shape. But where the Union of the contiguous Grains was more firm, the Divulsion there occasioned a larger Chasm, as at *b, b, b*

Some were also observed broken quite in two, and discovered by two different Substances, encompassing each other in the Manner of a White and Yolk, a nearer Resemblance still to Eggs, as *c, c, c.*

What we term the White, was pretty whitish near the Yolk, but grew more dusky towards the Shell, and in some was radiated like a *Pyrites*. The yolk-like Part was hollow in some, but filled in others with a darkish brown and porous Substance, like a Kind of Pitch, as at *d*

The *Interstices* or small Pores between the Globules, *e, e, e, e,* were found, b several Experiments, to be pervious every Way both to Air and Water, for on blowing through a Piece of this Stone of a considerable Thickness, the Air passed as easily as through a Cane. And when another pretty large Piece was covered all over with Cement, except at the two opposite Ends, by blowing in at one End, some Spittle wherewith the other was wetted, was raised into Abundance of Bubbles, and served to prove how porous some Bodies are which appear seemingly compact and close.

The Microscope discovers here a Stone, composed of innumerable minute Balls, which merely touch each other, and yet by so many Contacts constitute a Substance much harder than Free-Stone.

The Interstices between these Balls must render it very useful, when formed into proper Vessels, for the Filtration of Water or any other Liquors.

PLATE VI. FIG. 2.

A Sea-Moss.

THIS Picture represents a Kind of Sea-Plant or *Fucus*, called by Mr RAY, in his *Synopsis, Fucus telam lineam sericeamve texturâ suâ æmulans* It grows on the Rocks under Water, and spreads out into a great Tuft, which branches into several Leaves of a most beautiful and surprising Structure. But of this we shall defer giving any farther Description, till we come to the first *Figure* of the Eleventh *Plate*.

PLATE VI. FIG. 3.

A Piece of Spunge.

THE Texture of this Object is discovered by the Microscope to consist of innumerable, small, short, round Fibres, nearly of the same Bigness, jointed very curiously together in a Kind of Net-like Form. The Joints are most commonly where only

E   three

three Fibres meet, few of them being found composed of four : But neither of the three Fibres seems the Stock whereon the others grow, all being of the same Size, and conducing equally to form the Joint.   The Length of the Fibres between the Joints is, however, very irregular and different, the Distance between some Joints being ten or twelve times more than between others   So that the three Fibres make not equitriangular Figures, but meet in such a manner that their three Angles differ greatly from one another.   The Meshes or Holes of this reticulated Body are likewise extremely various, some having two, three, or four, others five, six, seven, eight, or nine Sides.   But of all these Particulars 'tis hoped the Picture will give a pretty good Idea.   Besides these microscopical Pores which lie between the Fibres, there are Multitudes of round Holes piercing from the Top of the Spunge into the Body thereof, and passing sometimes quite through it to the Bottom.

Dr. HOOKE observes, that Spunge is commonly reckoned as one of the *Zoopbyts* or *Plant-Animals*; which Opinion the Microscope confirms, by shewing the Contexture of it to be such as has been found in no other Vegetable   Different Ways of Trial prove likewise its Resemblance to Animal Substances , for examined chymically, it affords a volatile Salt and Spirit like Hartshorn ; when burnt in a Fire or at a Candle, it affords a fleshy Smell, not much unlike to Hair : And if we attempt to tear it or pull it asunder, the Strength and Toughness of its resisting Fibres prove them like the Fibres of Animals

BELLONIUS, in the Eleventh Chapter of his Second Book *de Aquatilibus*, informs us,
" That *Spunges* in the Sea are extremely different from what they are when dry, sticking
" to the Rocks, as many Species of the *Fungi* do to Trees, two or three Foot sometimes
" under the Sea-Water , tho' now and then not above four Inches.   Those Hollows
" which we see empty in *Spunges*, or in dry *Spunges* wash'd and wrung out, are filled,
" whilst on the Rocks, with a filthy Liquor, or rather Jelly-like Matter, which stinks
" enough to make one sick, even at a considerable Distance.   ARISTOTLE supposed
" them to have some kind of Life, from their Manner of fixing themselves to the
" Rocks, whence, says he, it is very difficult to pull them away, unless they are taken
" as it were by Surprize ; for at the Approach of any body to lay hold on them,
" they contract immediately, and fasten themselves so as not to be removed with-
" out a great deal of Trouble   They do the same likewise whenever there are
" Storms and Tempests.   The nasty Matter before mentioned may be supposed given
" them by Nature instead of Flesh, and the larger Cavities seem a Sort of Bowels or
" Intestines to them   The Part whereby they fasten to the Rocks, is like the Foot-
" Stalk of a Leaf, whence a slender Sort of Neck begins, which widening upwards,
" forms the globous Figure of the Head   On the Upper-Part almost all the Passages
" are hid by being closed, but four or five of them are open towards the Bottom, through
" which we may suppose their Nourishment is sucked in "

If a dry Spunge be thoroughly wetted, and then squeezing out the Water, it be suffered to expand itself into its natural Shape and Dimensions, which it will freely do whilst moist, 'tis very plain that the Mouths of the larger Holes have a kind of Lip or Rising round about them.   'Tis also evident, that each of these great Passages has many smaller ones below that help to constitute it, as many little Streams contribute to the making up a large River

In short, the Texture of *Spunge* is wonderful, and if it be properly examined into, seems to promise some Information of the Vessels hitherto undiscovered in Animal Substances, by reason the Solidity of the interserted Flesh in them is not easily removed, without destroying also those interspersed Vessels .   Whereas the *Parenchyma*, or what serves instead of Flesh to *Spunge*, is but a Kind of Jelly, easily cleared and washed away.

The Natural History of this Production is so imperfectly known, that we are still uncertain whether it increases from little to great like Vegetables, that is, Part after Part , or like Animals, all the Parts growing equally together .   Whether it affords *Matrices* or *Nests* for some Kinds of Water-Animals, or is a real Animal itself; and also, whether at any time it is more soft and tender, or of another Nature and Configuration

As the Discovery of the *Polype* has set many curious Gentlemen both in *France* and *England* upon a strict Examination of the Waters and their Productions, 'tis to be hoped that all these Doubts will shortly be cleared up.

An

The Pores of Charcoal p.15   Plate VII
Fig 1.

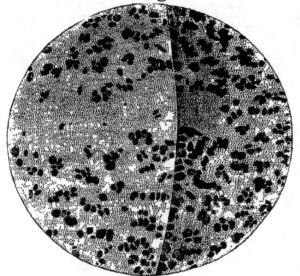

Pores of Petrifyed Woods p.15
Fig 2.

An EXPLANATION of the SEVENTH PLATE.

FIG. 1.

A Piece of Charcoal.

A Piece of Stick charred or burnt till it becomes black *, if broke short between the Charcoal
Fingers, appears with a shining smooth Surface, resembling the Surface of black
Sealing-Wax, which examined by a small Magnifier, exhibits Abundance of such Pores
as are visible to the naked Eye in many Kinds of Wood, ranged round the Pith as well
circularly as radiating from a Center These appear every where in the Substance of the
Coal, drilling it from End to End, so that you may easily blow through it.

But besides these many great and irregular Spots or Pores, if a Glass that magnifies
much be made use of, an infinite Number of exceedingly small and very regular Pores
will be discovered, so thick, so orderly set, and so close to one another, that very little
Room is left between them to be occupied by a solid Body, for the intermediate Partitions of these Pores appear so thin in some Places, that a Honey-comb is not less solid,
tho' in others they are much thicker, in proportion to the Holes

The exceeding Smallness and Closeness of these Pores may be conceived in some degree
by their Numbers, for no less than one hundred and fifty of them were counted in a Line
not more than the eighteenth Part of an Inch long, consequently, a Line of an Inch in
Length must contain two thousand seven hundred of them. and about five Millions seven
hundred twenty five thousand three hundred and fifty of the like Pores must be in a *circular
Area* of an Inch Diameter. Nay, *Cocus, black* and *green Ebony, Lignum Vitæ, Guaja-
cum,* &c. have their Pores still smaller, and more numerous; so exquisite are the Pipes
or Sluices whereby the Juices of Vegetables are conveyed !

PLATE VII. FIG. 2.

A Piece of petrified Wood.

THE Pores in this Object were not so much bigger than those in the foregoing Fi- Petrified
gure, as the Draught before us shews them; for this was viewed by a Microscope Wood
that magnified six times more than what was used for the Piece of Charcoal, and the
Drawing made in the same Proportion. Each Pore, however, was nearly half as large
again as those in the burnt Wood, and the Disposition of the whole exactly in the same
Figure and Order as the small Pores of Charcoal, but there were none of the larger Pipes
or Cavities before described in that.

The Subject under Examination seemed to have been a Part of some large Tree, that
had been broken off by Rottenness, before it became petrified. And Dr. HOOKE declares,
that all he had seen of this Kind seemed to have been rotten before the Petrifaction began.
and that he was confirmed in this Opinion, by examining a vast large Oak, which with mere
Age was rotten as it stood, whose Wood in Colour, Grain, and Shape, appeared exactly
like this petrified Substance. He likewise observes, that all those *microscopical Pores*, which
in sappy and sound Wood are filled with the natural Juices of the Tree, were found in
this (when viewed with magnifying Glasses) empty, like those of Charcoal, but much
larger than any he had seen in Charcoal.

Pieces of petrified Wood are however very different in Shape, Colour, Grain, Texture, and Hardness, some being brown and reddish, others grey like an Hone, some
black, flint-like, hard and brittle, others soft like a Slate or Whetstone.

In this Petrifaction the Parts seemed not at all altered from their Position whilst Wood,
having the Pores of Wood still remaining, with a manifest Difference between the Grain
and Bark; but it differed from Wood in Weight, Hardness, Closeness, Incombustible-
ness, and Brittleness

Its Weight was to common Water as Three and a Quarter to One, whereas few
English Woods, when very dry, are quite equal in Weight to Water.

It

* For the Manner of Charring Coal, *vid,* EVELYN's *Sylva,* p. 100, 101, 103

2

It was nearly as hard as Flint, and refembled the Grain thereof in fome Parts, would eafily cut Glafs, could fcarcely be fcratched itfelf by a black hard Flint, and would as readily as any common Flint ftrike Fire againft a Steel.

Its Clofenefs was evident when placed in fome Pofitions, for the Reafon why the Pores appeared darker than the reft of the Body, was then fhewn, *viz.* becaufe they were filled with a darker Subftance, and not becaufe they were hollow

Though kept fome time red-hot in the Flame of a Lamp, rendered very intenfe by a Blow-Pipe and a large **Charcoal**, it loft nothing of its Subftance, but appeared as folid as before, only fomewhat darker. 'Twas remarkable that it foon grew red-hot, and neither confumed like Wood, nor cracked and flew like Flint.

Diftilled Vinegar being dropped upon it, many fuch Bubbles were raifed inftantly, as are obfervable when it corrodes Corals.

It was fo brittle that one Blow of a Hammer would break off a Piece, and two or three more reduce it to a Powder.

It felt alfo much colder than Wood, and much like other clofe Stones and Minerals.

An EXPLANATION of the EIGHTH PLATE.

FIG. 1.

The Pores in Cork.

Cork

THE Circular Figure we are now defcribing, exhibits two of the thinneft Slices of Cork that could be fhaved off with a Penknife, made as fharp as poffible, in order to difcover, by the Microfcope, the Texture and Form thereof And, upon Examination, they were found to be all cellular or porous, in the Manner of an Honey-comb, but not fo regular The folid Subftance was alfo very fmall, in Comparifon of the Cavities, for the Partition between the Cells were near as thin in Proportion to them, as the flender Divifions in an Honey-comb are in Proportion to the Cells they feparate.

The Cells of Cork are ranged like fo many Rays tending from the Center or Pith of the Tree outwards · They are not very deep, but refemble many little Boxes, made by Numbers of Partitions dividing one long continued Pore, as is fhewn by the Slice marked B, which being a transverfe Section, prefents a View of the Pores opened lengthwife.

The Slice marked A, was fhaved off the long Way of the Cork, and confequently fhews all the Pores cut afunder transverfely, but the folid Partitions between them appeared not fo thick as they are here reprefented.

Several of thefe Lines being numbered, about Threefcore of the fmall Cells, placed end-ways, were found, ufually, in the Length of the eighteenth Part of an Inch wherefore the Length of an Inch muft contain above a Thoufand, a fquare Inch above a Million, or 1,166,400, and a cubic Inch above twelve hundred Millions, or 1,259,712,000; a thing almoft incredible, did not our Microfcope affure us of it by ocular Demonftration.

This Contexture, difcoverable by the Microfcope, proves the Lightnefs, of Cork to proceed, as it does in *Wool, Spunge, Pumice-Stone*, &c from its having a very fmall Quantity of folid Matter, extended into exceeding large Dimenfions. It proves likewife, that its Unaptnefs to fuck in, and confequently its floating on the Surface of Water, is owing to its whole Subftance being almoft filled with Air, inclofed in thofe innumerable little Cells or Boxes above defcribed, which being full already, are impenetrable to Water or other Air. Its Springingnefs, its Ability of being compreffed into half the Dimenfions it occupied before, and its Power of extending itfelf into the fame Space, when fuffered to act again, may likewife be accounted for from the fame Caufes. It is alfo probable that the Sides of, and Partitions between the Cells, may have in them an elaftic Quality, as moft Kinds of Vegetable Subftances have, and fo help to reftore themfelves to their former Pofition.

Common as Cork is, its Production is known but little, and therefore it may not be unacceptable to give a fhort Account thereof

In the South Parts of *France*, in *Spain* and *Italy*, there are feveral Species of what they call the *Cork-Tree* But the broad-leaved Sort, that is ever green, and affords the moft and beft Cork, is a pretty tall Tree, bearing Acorns like an Oak, tho' with Leaves much

larger

Plate VIII

Pores of Cork in two different Sections p 16

Fig I.

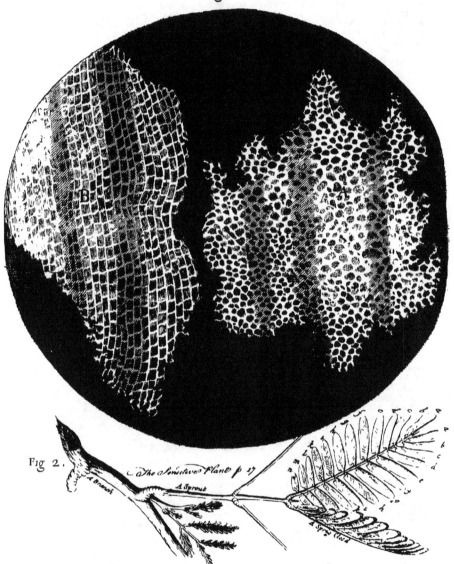

Fig 2.

The Sensitive Plant p 17

A Branch

A Sprout

larger and longer, fofter, and of a lighter green. Its Boughs are fewer, the Trunk bigger in proportion to its Height, and the Bark a great deal thicker, very light, fpungy, and of an Afh-colour, inclining towards a yellow, which Bark is the Cork.

Some *Naturalifts* imagine this Cork to be only an Excrefcence, or Subftance diftinct from the Tree itfelf, tho' drawing its Nourifhment therefrom, like *Ivy, Agaric,* and feveral Species of *Fungi*, which Opinion they ground on its having two Barks lying under it, in common to all Trees, on the Cork-Tree's being of fome Growth before this Subftance comes to be difcernable, on its cracking, flawing, and cleaving into many great Pieces, while the two Barks underneath remain entire, and on its being feparated and removed from the Tree, without doing it the leaft Injury, but on the contrary rendering it more vigorous and flourifhing Whereas, if not taken away in a certain Time, it either cracks and falls off itfelf, or elfe deftroys the Tree

People that prepare this Subftance for Sale, make a perpendicular Incifion through the Length of the whole Tree, and two Incifions tranfverfely, one towards the Top, and the other at the Bottom of the Trunk Then carefully clearing off the Cork, without it being fhattered, in large and even Pieces, which renders it of more Value, they foak it in Water, loading it with Weights to keep it down, and when fufficiently wetted, lay it over burning Coals (whereby its Outfide becomes blackened) to reduce it to a Flatnefs, and afterwards, to preferve this Flatnefs, they place it on an exact Level, heaping great Stones upon it. When perfectly dry, it is made up in Bales for Tranfportation *Johnfion* tells us, that the internal Part of the Cork-Tree is fo clofe and folid it will not fwim in Water, and that in three Years after the Cork has been cleared away, it will be overgrown with another fuch-like Covering

A Structure fimilar to this difcovered by the Microfcope in *Cork*, is likewife to be found in the Pith of Elder, or almoft any other Tree, and alfo in the Stalks of feveral other Vegetables, as *Fennel, Hemlock, Carrots, Teafels, Fern, Daucus, Burdock, Rufhes,* fome Kinds of *Reeds,* &c. but however with this Difference, that the Pores in thefe are ranged the long Way of the Stalk, whereas in *Cork* they run tranfverfe

PLATE VIII. FIG. 2.

The Senfible Plant.

THE Figure here given is intended to illuftrate the Obfervations made by Dr HOOKE, *Auguft* 9th, 1661, on the *Humble* and *Senfible Plants* then growing in Mr. CHIFFIN's Garden, St. *James's Park*, in the Prefence of Lord BROUNKER, Sir ROBERT MORAY, Dr WILKINS, Mr. EVELYN, and Dr CLARK

There were four Plants of the *Senfitive* Kind, two of which the Doctor diftinguifhes by the Name of the *Humble Plant,* becaufe in them, when the Leaves had clofed themfelves together, either by being gently touched, or if the Sun fhine very warm, by only taking off the Glafs that covered them, the tender Sprouts, as if withei'd, hung downwards to the Ground

They were little Shrub-Plants, having a fhort Stock, that rofe about an Inch above the Earth, from which feveral Branches iffued, round, ftrait, and fmooth, but with a Couple of fharp thorny Prickles juft under each of the Sprouts that proceeded from them

The Diftance between the Sprouts was ufually fomething above an Inch, and the End of each Sprout had generally four Sprigs, two at the Extremity, and one on each Side juft under it On each of thefe Sprigs, from its uppermoft Side, about eleven Pair of Leaves grew out, one againft another exactly, and neatly fet, in fuch-like Articulations as when the round Head of a Bone is received into a Socket that affords it an eafy Motion The Leaves were placed in the moft proper Manner to fold together readily, and when they clofed in Pairs, each Under-Pair folded a little over that above it, as the Picture fhews, where the Sprig is reprefented clofed.

Each Leaf, being almoft an oblong Square, grew out from the Sprig at one of the lower Corners, and received therefrom not only a Spine, (if we may fo call it) which paffed through and divided it lengthways, in fuch a Manner, that the Out-fide was broader than the Inner, but alfo fmall Fibres, paffing obliquely towards the oppofite broader Side, and feeming to render it a little mufcular, in order to move the whole Leaf All the Leaves and Sprigs were covered with fmall whitifh Hairs

On touching any of the Sprigs, all the Leaves on that Sprig contracted themfelves by Pairs, and joined their upper Surfaces clofe together

On letting a Drop of *Aqua-fortis* fall on the Sprig, between the Leaves *f f,* all the Leaves above, as *a, b, c, d, e,* fhut themfelves prefently, thofe below, as *g, h, i, k, l, m, n,* did the fame afterwards, by Pairs, fucceffively. Soon after the fame Motion began in the

F

the lower Leaves of the other Branches, which closed together in Pairs to the End of each Sprig, with some little Distance of Time betwixt But, next Day, all the Leaves were spread out again on the other Sprigs; on the Sprig where the *Aqua-fortis* had been dropped, the Leaves, downwards, were also expanded, green, and closing upon the Touch, though all above *ff*, were dead and wither'd.

One of the Leaves, *b b*, was clipped off in the Middle with a Pair of Scissars, as quick as it could be done; whereupon that Pair, and the Pair above it closed instantly, as did after a little Interval *d d, e e*, and all the other Pairs to the Bottom of the Sprig The Motion then began in the lower Leaves on the other Sprigs, and they shut themselves also, by Pairs, upwards, though not with such distinct Distances

These Plants were so extremely *sensible*, that their Leaves closed at the *Effluvia* of a strong-scented Oil, and likewise at the Smoak of Sulphur. The Sun-Beams had also the same Effect.

On cutting off a little Sprout, there issued from the Part whence it was cut, two or three Drops of a clear bright greenish Liquor, tasting somewhat bitterish at first, but leaving afterwards a Taste like Liquorice

A Sprig whose Leaves were all shut, being plucked off, with Design to observe the Liquor should come from it, none, even with pressing, could be found therein. Whereupon another Sprig, whose Leaves were expanded, being pulled off as dexterously as possible, upon the closing of the Leaves, a little of the forementioned Liquor was obtained from the End of the Sprig This Experiment was tried twice, (which was as often as the Plant could be robbed without Danger of killing it) and succeeded both Times in the same Manner

The Doctor imagines a constant Communication between every Part of this Plant and its Root, either by a Circulation of this Liquor, or a constant Pressure of its subtiler Parts to every Extremity of the Plant, and that the Motion and Closing of its Leaves are occasioned by some Impediment, which the Touch of any Thing produces in such Circulation or Pressure of the more subtile Parts of this Liquor. The Manner after which he supposes this to be effected, is too long and inconclusive to be inserted here

He says, the other two Plants never flagged, or hung down their Branches, nor shut their Leaves, but upon somewhat of a hard Stroke Their Stalks grew up from the Root, and were more herbaceous, being round and smooth, without any Prickles The Sprouts from them had several Pair of Sprigs, with seventeen Pair of Leaves (much smaller than these on the *Humble-Plant)* most commonly on each Sprig

There are many Species of the *Sensitive Plant*, that differ much in Size, Figure, and Degree of Sensibility We are told, that in the Passage of the *Isthmus*, from *Nombre de Dios* to *Panama*, there is a Wood of *Sensitive Trees*, the Leaves of which, as soon as they are touched, move with a rattling Noise, and close, and twist themselves together into a winding Figure

Plate IX

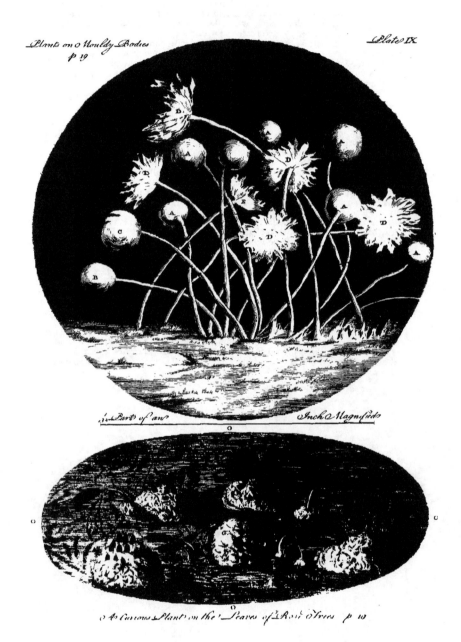

The 32 Part of an   Inch Magnified.

A Curious Plant on the Leaves of a Rose Trees p 19

An EXPLANATION of the NINTH PLATE.

FIG. 1.

The Form of Blue or White Mould

FRUITS, Herbs, Leaves, Roots, Cheeſe, Leather, and many other moiſt Things, are Mouldineſs frequently obſerved with hairy Spots upon them, of a blue or white Colour, ſuch as we commonly call *Mouldineſs* The Figure now before us was a Spot of that Kind, found on the red Sheep-ſkin Cover of a Book, and examined by the Microſcope, which diſcovered it to be a pretty Sort of Vegetable, puſhing out Multitudes of ſmall long cylindrical and tranſparent Stalks, not exactly upright, but bending a little with the Weight of a round white Knob or Ball, that grew on the Top of each

Many of theſe Knobs were very round, and had a ſmooth Surface, ſuch as A A A A A A
Others were alſo ſmooth, but ſomewhat of an oblong Shape, as B
Several of them were broken a little, appearing with a few Clefts on the Top, as C
Others again were ſhattered, or flown to pieces, in the Manner of D D D D.

Their whole Subſtance was very tender, much like that of the ſofter Kind of common white Muſhroom, for the leaſt Touch with a Pin tore them, and though they grew near together in a Cluſter, each Stem ſeemed to riſe from a ſeparate Root, out of a diſtinct Part or Pore of the Leather.   Some were ſmall and ſhort, ſeeming but newly ſprung up, with Balls for the moſt part round.   Others were taller and larger, being probably of a longer Growth, the Heads of which appeared moſtly broken, and ſeveral of them much waſted, as E

It was not eaſy to find out what theſe Heads contained, or whether they were Flowers or Seed-Veſſels ; but they ſeemed to bear the neareſt Reſemblance to the Heads of Muſhrooms, and were very diſagreeable both to the Taſte and Smell

The Microſcope diſcovers ſeveral Species of minute Plants, very different from one another, compoſing what we call Mouldineſs, as found on different Sorts of Things, and at different Seaſons of the Year , ſome reſemble Spunge, others Puff-Balls, and others a Thicket of Buſhes, very much branched, and extending much in Length, in proportion to their Thickneſs, like creeping Brambles.

Our Author ſuppoſes that *Muſhrooms*, and the *Microſcopical Plants*, we are now deſcribing, may be generated at any Time, and from any Kind of putrified Subſtance, either animal or vegetable, without Seed , merely by the friendly Concurrence of either natural or artificial Heat and Moiſture   And adds, that he could never find any thing like Seeds in *Muſhrooms* But later Diſcoveries have proved him greatly miſtaken in this Reſpect, by ſhewing that *Muſhrooms* produce Seeds in prodigious Numbers, as any Body may be ſatisfied who will take the Trouble to examine the Gills of them with good Glaſſes · And tho' it may be impoſſible to diſcern the like on theſe minute Plants, it is not improbable that their round Heads may contain alſo an Abundance of Seeds, which becoming ripe in a few Hours, are ſpirted to ſome ſmall Diſtance round about, where finding a proper Bed, they preſently ſpring up, and ſoon bear Seeds themſelves

And if ſo, we need no longer wonder at the ſpeedy ſpreading of Mouldineſs over any Body whereon it once appears.   It muſt be owned, that Heat and Moiſture, and oftentimes a Degree of Putrefaction in the Subſtance, are requiſite to make theſe little Plants thrive , but that ſuch Principles ſhould be able to create them, muſt, I think, be paſt the Belief of any who have ſtudied Nature by the Help of Glaſſes.

PLATE IX.   FIG 2.

A curious Plant on the Leaves of Roſe-Trees.

TOwards the End of Summer, when the Leaves of *Damaſk-Roſe* Trees begin to Plants Roc dry and turn yellow, they frequently have yellow Specks on their upper Surface, free Lev over againſt which, exactly on the Under-ſide, may be found little yellow Hillocks of a gummy Subſtance, with black Specks in the Middle of them, appearing to the naked Eye no bigger than the ſmalleſt Tittle that can be made with a Pen

The Oval Figure O O O O, which is given here, as examined by the Microſcope, was a Piece of *Roſe-Leaf*, about the Size of the little Oval marked X, on the Hillock C. On

i   the

this appeared feveral Knobs of a yellowifh red gummy Subftance, out of which fprung Multitudes of long Pods, in Shape refembling thofe of common Mofs, but, fo much lefs, that many Hundreds of them would not be equal to one Seed-Pod of Mofs The Stalks whereon they grew were finely tranfparent, and almoft like the Stalks of the Plants in *Mouldinefs,* but fomewhat yellower.

Some of thefe Hillocks appeared barren or deftitute, without any thing growing on them, as G

The Pods in others, were juft fhooting out their Heads, and feemed all pointing directly upwards, as at A

In fome, as at B, they were juft gotten out of the Hillock, with Pods of an indifferent Size, but little or no Stalk

They were found in fome beginning to have little fhort Stalks, as C.

In others, as D, the Stalks were increafed both in Length and Thicknefs

Others ftill, as E, F, H, I, K, L, produced Pods and Stalks that were a great deal larger, and probably at their full Growth: The Stalks were more bulky about the Root, and tapering towards the Top, as F and L moft particularly fhew.

No Seeds could be difcovered in thefe Pods, but as they grew to their full Size they began to bend their Heads downward, in the Manner thofe of common Mofs do, whereby Nature feems to intend the fame as in many Seed Veffels of greater Bulk, *viz* that the Seed, when ripe, fhould be fhaken and fcattered out at the Ends of them, as we fee it is in the *Columbine,* &c.

If thefe Pods, as is highly probable, contain Seeds, and the Size of thofe Seeds bears fuch a Proportion to that of the Pod, as we find between the Seeds and Seed Veffels of *Pinks, Columbines, Poppies,* &c how inconceivably minute muft each of thofe Seeds be! The whole Length of one of the largeft Pods was not the five hundredth Part of an Inch, and in fome not above the thoufandth Part, certainly therefore many thoufand fuch Seeds muft be neceffary to conftitute a Bulk vifible to the naked Eye, and, if each of thefe contains the Rudiments of a young Plant of the fame Kind, what muft we think of the conftituent Parts, Sap-veffels, and Pores thereof?

❁❁❁❁❁❁❁❁❁❁❁❁❁❁❁❁❁❁❁❁❁❁❁❁❁❁❁❁❁❁❁❁❁❁❁❁❁❁

An EXPLANATION of the TENTH PLATE.

Small Wall-Mofs

Wall Mofs
THIS Plate exhibits the different Parts of a fmall and beautiful, but very common Species of *Mofs,* as they appeared before the Microfcope

The Root A refembles a feedy Parfnep, furnifhed with fmall Strings and Fibres, finely branched, like the Roots of much larger Vegetables From this the Body of the Plant fprings up, of a Shape fomewhat quadrangular, moft curioufly fluted with little Hollows running parallel all its Length Its Sides are clofely fet with a Multitude of large, fur, well fhaped Leaves, fome rounder, and others longer, according to their Age, as B, C

When this Plant is young, and fpringing up as C, 'tis not unlike to *Houfeleek,* having fuch kind of thick Leaves, folding over one another, but when they grow longer, the Surface on each Side of them becomes beautifully covered with little oblong tranfparent Bodies, as the Leaves D, D, D, exprefs

There fhoots out between the Leaves, a fmall white tranfparent hair-like Body, which becomes in time a long, round, and even Stalk, as E, which being cut tranverfely, when dry, was found to be a ftuff, hard, and hollow Cane or Reed, without any kind of Knot or Joint, from its Bottom, where the Leaves furrounded it, to the Top where a large Seed-Cafe grew.

F reprefents the Seed-Veffel or Cafe, cut off from the Stalk E, and covered with a thin whitifh Skin G, terminating in a long thorny Top This fkinny Membrane at firft inclofes the whole Seed-Veffel, but as that fwells within it, the fkin breaks by degrees, and at length falls off with its thorny Top, leaving the Seeds to ripen, and be fcattered from an Opening, to be defcribed prefently, which before was covered by it

H fhews the Seed-Veffel, when ripe, without its membranous Covering G The Top hereof before the Seeds are ripe appears like a flat burr'd Button I, and has no Hole or Opening, but as they ripen, the Button grows bigger, and a round Hole K opens itfelf exactly in the Center, through which the Seed is fhed And for the more readily effecting

i

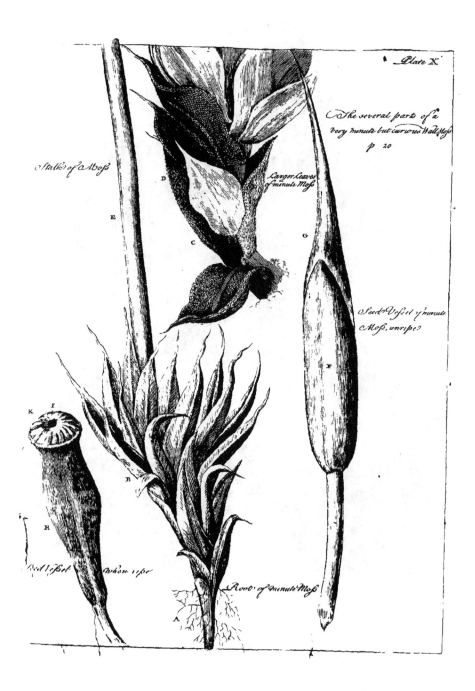

Plate X.

The several parts of a
very minute but curious Wall Moss
p 20

Stalks of Moss

Larger Leaves
of minute Moss

Seed Vessel of minute
Moss, unripe

Roots of minute Moss

Seed Vessel, when ripe

Plate XI

The Configuration of a beautiful Sea Moss, whereof the whole Figure is given. Plate VI

Fig. I p. 22

The Eight   of an Inch

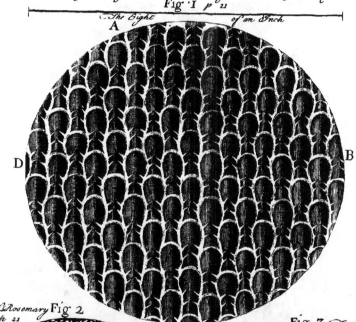

A

D   B

C

Piece of Rosemary Fig 2   Fig. 3 Fine Lawn p. 22
Leaf p. 22

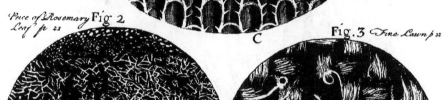

this, Nature wonderfully difpofes this End of the Cafe to bend itfelf downwards, as the Ears of Wheat and Barley ufually do when ripe.

On opening fome of thefe Cafes, when dry and red, they were found quite empty; but being cut afunder with a fharp Pen-knife, while green, a fmaller round Cafe was difcovered within the other, with a Multitude of ftringy Fibres, occupying the Space between the two Cafes, the innermoft whereof was full of exceedingly minute white Seeds, as in the Seed-Veffel of a *Carnation*, after the Flowers have been a few Days fallen off

Our Author compares the Thicknefs of this little Vegetable, with that of fome Trees we have Accounts of in the hot Climates of *Guinea* and *Brazil*, (the Bodies of which are, they tell us, twenty Feet in Diameter, whereas the Body of this Mofs is, commonly, not more than the fixtieth Part of an Inch), and finds, by Calculation, that the Thicknefs of the one exceeds that of the other 2,985,984 Millions of Times. He then fuppofes the Production on a Rofe-Leaf, juft now defcribed, to be a thoufand Times lefs bulky than this Mofs, and, confequently, that one of thefe Trees muft exceed the Bulk of that a thoufand Times the Number above given. So prodigioufly various are the Works of the Creator! and fo all-fufficient his Power to perform what to Man would feem impoffible.

An EXPLANATION of the ELEVENTH PLATE.

FIG. 1.

A Piece of Sea-Weed.

THE Subject under our Eye at prefent, is a fmall Piece, (the eighth Part of an Inch only in Diameter) of a moft beautiful *Fucus* or *Sea-Wrack*, a large Tuft whereof is given, *Fig.* 2 *Plate* VI very little bigger than its natural and common Size, but the Piece we are now defcribing, A, B, C, D, is magnified a great deal. The whole Surface of this Plant appears covered with a moft curious Kind of carved Work, confifting of a Texture much refembling Honey-comb, and feems every where full of innumerable Holes, no bigger than what the Point of a fmall Pin would make, ranged in the Manner of a *Quincunx*, or like the pearled Rows in the Eye of a Fly, which are exactly regular which way foever they are obferved.

These little Holes, which the naked Eye would imagine circular, are fhewn by the Microfcope to be of quite a different Figure, having nearly the Shape of the Sole of a round-toed Shoe, the hinder Part whereof feems covered, as it were, by the Toe of the next that follows it Each Hole is edged about with a very thin and tranfparent Subftance, of a pale Straw-Colour, from which four fmall tranfparent Thorns, of the fame Colour, iffue, two on each Side, and almoft meet acrofs the Cavity But no Words can give fo good a Notion of fuch a wonderful and uncommon Structure as the Picture now before us.

This Species of Sea-Weed is called by Mr. RAY, *Fucus telam lineam fericeanrve textura fua æmulans*, by others, the *broad-leaved horned Wrack*. It is found here and there, thrown by the Sea upon the Shores; but as no body has ever feen it growing, it is probably produced in the deepeft Parts thereof.

The Sea affords an endlefs Variety of Corals, Corallines, Spunges, Moffes, &c. every Part of which is a delightful Object for the Microfcope.

PLATE XI. FIG. 2.

A Piece of Rofemary-Leaf.

THE Under-fide of the Leaf was what Dr. HOOKE examined, and what, he fays, exhibited to him a fmooth and fhining Surface. A B, is a Part of the Upper-fide of the Leaf, but by a kind of Doubling turns down and covers fome of the Under-fide, looking like a quilted Bag of green Silk, or like fome very pliable and tranfparent Membrane filled out with a green Liquor Several other Plants have Leaves, whofe Sur-

G faces

faces are fmooth like this, and as it were quilted, in the fame manner. Rue, or Herb-graff, is polifhed, and all over indented or pitted.

The Part that might properly be called the Under fide of the Leaf, had a downy Sur-face, which appeared through the Microfcope much like a Thicket of Bufhes.

The Leaves and Stalks of moft Vegetables are covered with Down or Hair, and there feems as great a Variety in the Shape, Size, and Growth of thefe fecundary Plants, (if we may fo term them, being fomewhat analagous to the Hairs in Animals) as there is be-tween fmall Shrubs   They confift ufually of fmall tranfparent Parts, fome in the Form of minute Needles, as on the *Thiftle*, *Cowage*, *Nettle*, &c   Others are like Cats-Claws, as the Hooks of *Clivers*, the Beards of *Barley*, the Edges of feveral Sorts of *Grafs*, *Reeds*, &c.   And on many Plants, fuch as Colts-foot, Rofe-Campion, Poplar, Willow, and all the downy Kinds, they grow in the Form of Bufhes, but much diverfified in each particular Plant

A Multitude of fmall round Balls, exactly globular, and much refembling Pearls, were obfervable amongft the little Bufhes or Down, as they are reprefented, C C C C C, &c.

Infinite Numbers of fuch as thefe may be difcerned on *Sage* and feveral other Plants; which was probably the Reafon why KIRCHER fuppofed them covered with Spiders Eggs, though in truth thefe are nothing elfe but a kind of gummy Exfudation, and not the Eggs of any Infect, as may be concluded from their being found upon them all the Year, and fcarce changing their Magnitude at all.

D D D reprefent the irregular Difpofition of the downy or bufh-like Subftance.

PLATE VI. FIG. 3.

Fine Lawn.

THIS Object is a Piece of the fineft *Lawn*, as it appears before the Microfcope. It feems introduced by Miftake into this *Plate*, and belongs properly to *Plate* II. where *Ribbon*, *Taffaty*, and Things of its own Kind are examined.   A Defcription of it is therefore given where that Plate is explained, *Page* 4, to which we refer the Reader.

❀❀❀❀❀❀❀❀❀❀❀❀❀❀❀❀❀❀❀❀❀❀❀❀❀❀❀❀❀❀❀❀❀❀❀❀❀❀

An EXPLANATION of the TWELFTH PLATE.

FIG. 1.

A Piece of Stinging Nettle.

A Piece of *Stinging Nettle*, as enlarged by the Microfcope, is the Object now before us

The whole Surface of the Leaf is fet thick with fharp Thorns or Prickles, which are juft vifible to the naked Eye, but when magnified by Glaffes, their Form is difcoverable as at A B, A B, &c.   Each of thefe confifts of two Parts, different in Shape and Quality. The Part A refembles a round Bodkin, tapering from B, till it ends in a very fharp Point. Its Subftance is hard and ftiff, exceeding tranfparent, and hollow from Top to Bottom, as has been found by many Trials.   The lower and thicker Part B, which is as it were the Bafis whereon the Prickle ftands, and of a much more pliable Confiftence, in Shape re-fembles a wild Cucumber, and is evidently a little Bladder, or Veffel filled with a limpid Liquor, always in Readinefs to be ejected through the Cavity of the Prickle, when any thing preffes hard upon it

This Configuration enables us to account for the Effects of what we call the *Stinging of a Nettle*, the Manner of which the Doctor fully difcovered by the following curious Experiment.

Having provided a fingle Glafs, whofe *Focus* was at the Diftance of about half an Inch, faften'd in a little Frame, that it might be managed eafily, he perceived by the Help thereof, that on thrufting his Finger gently againft the Ends of a Nettle's Prickles, they did not bend in the leaft, but he could difcern a Liquor rifing towards the Points thereof,

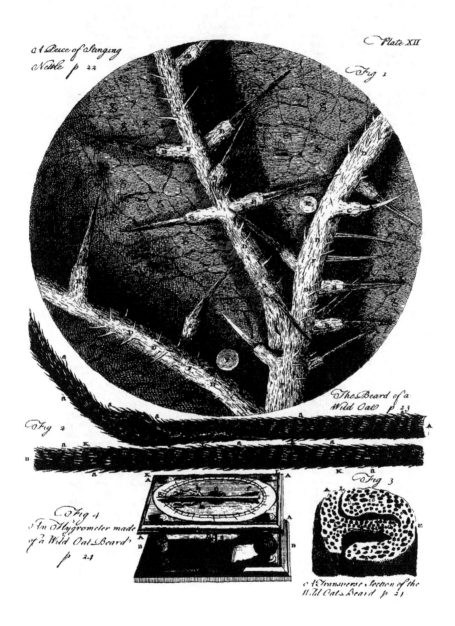

A Peice of Stinging
Nettle p 22

Plate XII

Fig 1

The Beard of a
Wild Oat p 23

Fig 2

Fig 3

Fig 4
An Hygrometer made
of a Wild Oat Beard
p 24

A Transverse Section of the
Wild Oats Beard p 24

thereof, or finking in them, according to the Degree of Preffure; and on taking away his Hand, he could fee it fubfide entirely into the little Bladder at the Bottom, and that as plainly as he had ever feen Water afcend and defcend in a Tube of Glafs.

A Prickle thus preffed upon, and the Liquor rifing in it, is reprefented by the Letter C

Hence it is evident to a Demonftration, that the burning acute Pain, Swelling and Inflammation that follow immediately on thrufting thefe Prickles into any Part of the Body, are owing to an Injection, at the fame Inftant, through the Cavities of thefe Prickles, of a corrofive or poifonous Juice, lodged in Bags or Bladders at the Roots of the faid Prickles, and forced to afcend in them by their being preffed down on the faid Bags or Bladders.

Such a Structure and Effect are exactly fimilar to the Sting of a *Scorpion, Wafp, Bee, &c* and the Confequence of being ftung thereby. For the Sting of thefe Animals, like the Thorn of a Nettle, is an exceeding fharp-pointed Tube, which entering the Skin or Flefh ferves to convey a poifonous Liquor into the Wound, that by irritating the nervous and fenfible Parts occafions all the enfuing Uneafinefs and Mifchief. And this Liquor, as in the Nettle, is prepared and contained in a little Bag at the Root or Bottom of the Sting. Nor is the Difference very great as to *Vipers* and other *Serpents,* whofe Bite is dangerous, for the Wounds their Teeth make would be very harmlefs, were they not hollow, and a Venom fquirted through them into the Wounds they give

D, D, D, D, *&c* are a Kind of Thorns or Prickles without any vifible Bladders of Liquor at their Roots, and a great deal fmaller, as well as more numerous, than thofe that have fuch Veffels Thefe probably may be no farther hurtful than to occafion a little Itching

F, E, a Sort of Pearl-like Globules, perfectly tranfparent, that are here and there interfperfed on both Sides the Leaf of this Plant, and grow to it much after the Manner as *Oak-Apples* grow on the Leaves of an Oak.

F, F, F, the Ribs or large Sap-Canals, whence all the Prickles iffue, and the Bladders at their Roots are conftantly fupplied with the pungent Juices they contain.

g g g g g g, &c are the intermediate and thinner Parts of the Leaf, which are almoft fmooth, and afford little remarkable, but an irregular Ramification of very fmall Veffels or Fibres.

PLATE XII. FIG. 2.

The Beard of a Wild-Oat.

THE Beard of a Wild-Oat, cut afunder at the Ends A and B, is reprefented by the two long prickly Figures we are now about to examine.

This little Production of Nature is wonderfully remarkable, on account of its making an exceeding good *Hygrometer,* or Inftrument for difcovering the *Drynefs* or *Moifture* of the Air, being extremely fenfibly of, and vifibly affected by the leaft Alteration as to thofe Particulars A Defcription of it muft therefore be an inftructive as well as entertaining Amufement.

To the naked Eye it appears very inconfiderable, being only a fmall black or brown Beard or Briftle, growing from the Side of the Inner-hufk that covers the Grain of a Wild-Oat. In *July* and *Auguft,* when the Grain is ufually ripe and dry, this Beard is bent fomewhat below the Middle almoft to a Right-Angle, and the under and thicker Part is writhed or twifted round down to the very Bottom, making three Revolutions in fome, in others more or lefs, according to the Bignefs and Maturity of the Grain whereon it grew, together with the Drynefs or Moifture of the ambient Air. It is very brittle when dry, and eafily broken from the Hufk from which it proceeds.

If it be put in Water, and viewed with a Magnifying-Glafs, it feems like a twifted *Withe,* having a Couple of Clefts or Channels along it, the fmall bent Top will then move round, the Under-Part untwift, and the Knee or Angle gradually become quite ftrait, in which Condition, being at full Length, it extends fometimes to an Inch and an half. When taken out of Water, and fuffered to dry again, it by Degrees twifts itfelf round as it was before, and bends again near the Middle into its former Pofture.

The Superficies of this little Body appears, by the Microfcope, adorned with little Channels and interjacent Ridges, ftrait where the Beard is not twifted, but writhed where it is Thefe Ridges are thickly befet on each fide with Prickles, not unlike the Quills of *Porcupines,* (as are fhewn by *a a a a a*) all the Points whereof are directed upwards towards the Top of the Beard, which is the Reafon it fticks and grates againft the Skin, if one endeavours to draw it between the Figures the contrary Way. The Manner of growing, Number, Clofenefs to each other, and Size of the Prickles, in proportion to the Beard, the Figure will alfo fhew

2   K K,

K K, in the upper Figure, reprefent the two Channels or Clefts opened, which reach from the Bottom to the Angle C, all along the writhed Part, and are twifted round with it, as at the Letters K K, &c. L L, &c. in both the Figures. Thefe Channels are filled up with a kind of fpungy Subftance.

PLATE XII. FIG. 3.

A tranfverfe Section of the Wild-Oat Beard.

ON cutting the twifted Part acrofs, to examine its Pith, with the Form and Difpofition of the Pores thereof, the Appearance was as A B C C E F.

K L reprefent the two Clefts or Channels, which as it were divide the Beard, its whole Length, into two unequal Parts, they wind very oddly in the inward Part of the Writhe.

C C fhew the Pores or Sap-Veffels running the long Way.

PLATE XII. FIG. 4.

An Hygrometer made with a Wild-Oat Beard.

A A, B B, is a Kind of Box or Frame, the Top and Bottom Plates whereof are held together only by four fmall Pillars, that a free Paffage for the Air between them may no ways be obftructed.

C is a fmall Hole in the Middle of the Under-Plate B B, into which Hole the Bottom of the Oat-Beard is fixed, upright, with foft *Bees-Wax*, in the Manner of *a b*, while the Upper-End thereof paffes through another Hole exactly oppofite in the Top-Plate A A A A.

On the Top of the Beard at *e*, a fmall and very light *Index*, *f g*, made of a thin Slip of *Reed* or *Cane*, muft be faftned with a Piece of fine Silk, or a Touch of hard Wax or Glue.

This Inftrument is fo extremely fenfible of the leaft Alteration in the Conftitution of the Air, as to Drynefs or Moifture, and does fo certainly twift or untwift itfelf in proportion thereto, that it will frequently untwift, and thereby turn the *Index* a whole Round, only by breathing on it, or twift and thereby turn it as much the contrary Way by letting it approach the Fire, or placing it in the Sun-fhine.

And becaufe, in Times of great Drynefs or Moifture, the *Index f g*, moves fometimes twice or thrice round, and may thereby make it difficult to form a right Judgment of it, the following Contrivance has been employed with good Succefs, to know certainly what Number of Revolutions have been made.

The *Index f g* being raifed to fome Diftance above the Surface of the Plate A A, a fmall Pin *b*, was fixed downwards pretty near the Middle of it, in fuch a manner that it might almoft touch the Surface of the Plate A A. And then another Pin being alfo fixed in a convenient Part of the faid Plate, whereon a fmall Piece of Paper, fhaped like the Figure *i k*, was placed, by making a Hole through its Center, which Paper having a convenient Number of Teeth, every Turn or Return of the Pin *b* moved its little indented Circle a Tooth forwards or backwards; whereby, as the Teeth were marked, it was eafy to afcertain how many Revolutions the *Index* made.

This little Circle may be made of thin Paftboard, Vellum, or Parchment, as well as Paper, but great Care muft be taken that it be exceeding light, and move very eafily upon the Pin, otherwife the whole Operation will be fpoiled. The Box may be made of Brafs, Silver, Iron, Wood, or Ivory, and Degrees marked upon it as every one chufes. and the *Index* may be contrived various Ways, to fhew not only the Number of Revolutions, but the minute Divifions of each.

BAPTISTA PORTA informs us, in his Book of *Natural Magic*, that fome *Jugglers*, by Means of the Beard of a Wild Oat, (which, to make it the more furprizing, they called the Leg of an *Arabian* Spider or an *Egyptian* Fly) ufed to make a fmall *Index*, Crofs, or the like, to move round, by putting a Drop of Water to it privately. though they pretended it was in Obedience to certain Words they muttered.

Twifted Cord, Cat-Gut, and fome other Things may be contrived to fhew the Changes as to Drought or Moifture in the Air, as well by ftretching and fhrinking, as by untwifting and twifting. But thefe are not near fo fenfible or exact, their varying Property alfo gradually diminifhes. The Beards of *Geranium Mofchatum*, and alfo of fome other Species of *Cranes-Bill*, are at leaft as eafily affected as that of the *Wild-Oat*. And it is farther obfervable, that the fmaller the writhing Subftance the quicker its Senfibility of every little Change.

Plate XIII

Seeds of Venus Looking Glass or Corn-Violet. p. 25

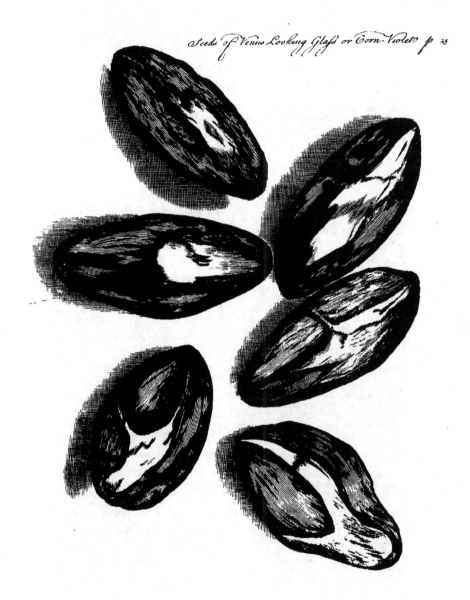

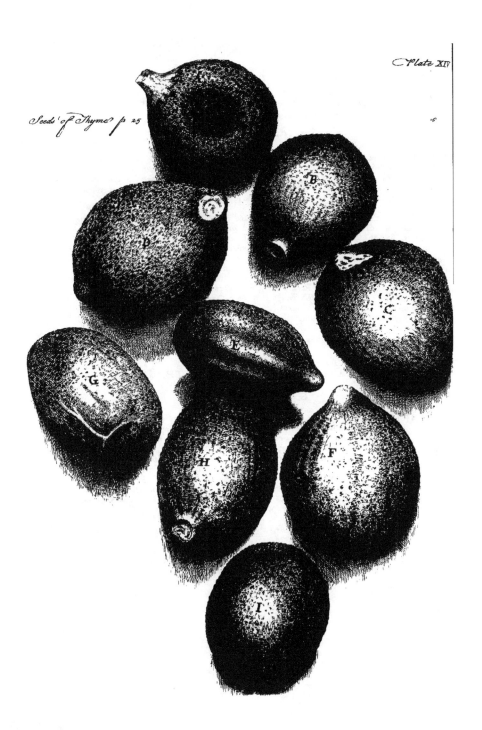

Plate XIV

Seeds of Thyme p 45

An EXPLANATION of the THIRTEENTH PLATE.

This and the Three following Plates *present to us the Pictures of different* Seed, *as they appear when enlarged by the* Microscope.

Seeds of the Corn-Violet.

THOSE under our Infpection, at prefent, belong to the *Corn-Violet*, or *Venus-* Looking-Glafs , whofe Seed is fmall, black and fhining ; and when feen by the naked Eye, refembles a little Flea , but magnified by Glaffes, appears in the Form before us, covered with a thick, tough and fhining Skin, fhrunk or pitted, as it were, irregularly, infomuch that no two of them can be found alike exactly *Seeds of the Corn-Violet*

The Seeds of Plants (even thofe whofe Shape and Structure, by reafon of their Smalnefs the Eye is unable to diftinguifh) are adorned with fuch a Variety of Carvings and Ornaments, that much Pleafure arifes from the Examination of them   Their Surfaces are fome curioufly wrought, others fmooth and polifhed ; fome are covered with Hairs, fome with a kind of Shell, and fome with both   Their mere outward Form renders them delightful Objects , but if we proceed farther, and by Diffection gain a Knowledge of their internal Structure, we fhall find ourfelves loft in a new World of Wonders   Dr. JAMES PARSONS, Fellow of the *Royal Society*, is at prefent engaged in thefe Difcoveries, which he propofes to lay before the Public , and as his Pencil is well qualified to delineate whatever his Eye obferves, there is great Reafon to expect from him an honeft and judicious Defcription of whatever is moft remarkable therein.

An EXPLANATION of the FOURTEENTH PLATE.

Seeds of Thyme.

NINE of the minute Seeds of *Thyme* are fhewn here, as they were magnified, and in different Pofitions both to the Eye and the Light.   There appeared a great Variety in their Bulk and Figure , but every one of them nearly refembled a Lemon or Orange dried, and that as well in Colour as Shape.   Some were a little rounder, and more like an Orange, as A, B, each whereof has a remarkable Part whereto their Stalks were joined , and on A a little Piece of Stalk is ftill remaining   The oppofite End of thefe Seeds has a Knob or Prominence, fuch as Lemons ufually have, which is fhewn by D, E, and F. *Thyme-Seeds*

They all feemed a little wrinkled or fhrivell'd, but the Seed H was moft remarkably fo. The Seed G had an irregular Ridge or Rifing, expreffed by the white Lines thereon. I reprefents a Seed nearly of an oval Shape.

An EXPLANATION of the FIFTEENTH PLATE.

Poppy-Seeds.

Poppy Seeds

THE Seeds of Poppy, when viewed by the Microscope, appear in Form very like a Kidney, with a pretty Kind of Net-work on them, rising in orderly Ridges above the Surface, and making hexagonal and pentagonal little Hollows, with Sides and Angles that are nearly regular.

They differ in Colour according to the Poppy producing them ; some Sorts are white, others of a dark-brownish red ; and the Seeds of a foreign Poppy commonly given to Birds by the Name of *Maw-Seed*, are very remarkable for being of a lightish-blue, which is a Colour found, perhaps, in no other Seeds.

" A Dust may be shaken from amongst the Seeds of Poppies, which looks very " agreeable when brought before the Microscope, having almost the same Appearances as " the Surfaces of the Seeds, with the Advantage of being transparent *   This Dust is " really the fine Membranes that lay between the Seeds, which, by the Pressure of the " Seeds against them, have received Marks corresponding to the Ridges and Hollows on " the Seeds themselves "

The Poppy-Heads, wherein the Seeds grow, are also well deserving our Observation, being round and regularly formed Bodies, with a most beautiful Crown on the Top of each, under the indented Projections whereof there are several Openings, when the Seeds become ripe, out of which they are scattered round about, as often as these Seed-Vessels are shaken by the Winds, or any other Accident.

The Seeds are disposed in many little Cells, divided each from other by fine Membranes, which reach, in an upright Position, from the Bottom of the Head to the Crown at its Top, all meeting at the Center : By which means every Cell is shaped like the Clove of a *China-Orange*, having at the Upper-End an Opening for the Seeds to scatter out at.

We should not shew a proper Regard for the Poppy, or pay a due Acknowledgment to the All-wise Dispenser of every Good, should we pass it over without taking notice of its singular Virtues.   For this only, amongst all the Productions of Nature, is capable of alleviating the racking Agonies of Pain, and producing comfortable and refreshing Sleep, when the Brain is overheated and the Spirits agitated almost to Madness   This therefore is one of the great Blessings Providence has bestowed on Man, and we greatly undervalue it, when we prefer the Grape, or any other Fruit or Plant before it ; since, in many Cases, this and this only can give Ease, without which not all the Mines of *India* can give Happiness.

Opium

In short, the milky Juice which flows from the green Heads or Seed-Vessels of the Poppy pretty freely upon cutting, after it becomes inspissated, is *Opium*.   A Drug esteem'd in the highest Manner in *Turky*, *Persia*, *India*, and all the Eastern Parts of the World, as it not only removes Grief and Pain, and produces an inexpressible Serenity and Satisfaction of Mind, but by the Help thereof the People of those Countries find themselves enabled to undergo the greatest Fatigues, and even to subsist without Food for several Days together.

The Goodness of Providence is therefore further observable in the Care it has taken for the abundant Propagation of this inestimable Vegetable ; the Seeds whereof it has made so small as not to exceed the thirty-second Part of an Inch in Diameter, whereas the Diameter of the Seed-Vessel is oftentimes two Inches, so that it is capable of containing near two hundred thousand Seeds ; and always does contain a prodigious Number. Every Root also produces several of these Seed-Vessels, the Contents of which together must amount to Millions.   This Plant is likewise found almost in every Country, and tho' its Virtues come far short in the colder Climates of what they are in the hotter, it may every where be made use of to good purpose

The Knowledge of *Opium*, and the Effects thereof, are probably of great Antiquity, for HOMER, the oldest Writer in the World except MOSES, describes HELEN preparing a Cordial called by him *Nepenthes*, whose Qualities and Effects agree admirably with

what

* *Microscope made easy*, p 254.

Plate X.

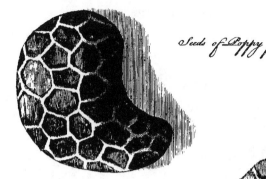

Seeds of Poppy p. 26

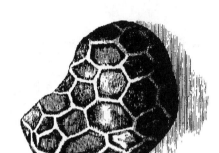

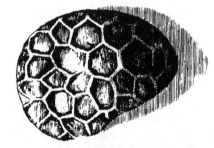

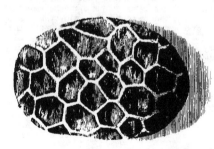

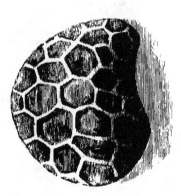

Plate XVI

Seeds of Purslain p 27

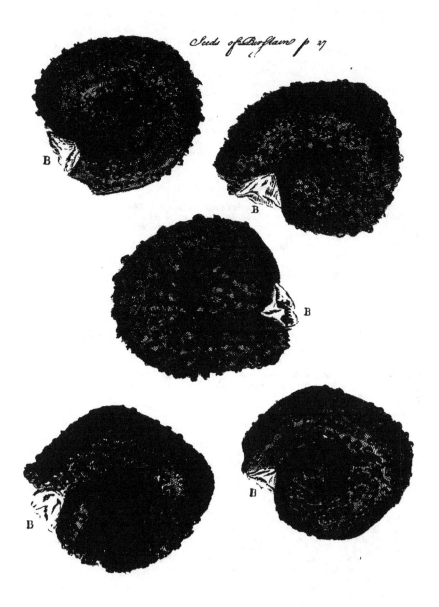

what we know of OPIUM. We ſhall therefore ſubjoin Mr POPE's excellent *Tranſlation* of that Paſſage from the Fourth Book of the ODYSSEY, *Line* 301

> - - - - *with genial Joy to warm the Soul*
> *Bright* HELEN *mix'd a Mirth-inſpiring Bowl*
> *Temper'd with Drugs of ſov'reign Uſe, t' aſſuage*
> *The boiling Boſom of tumultuous Rage ;*
> *To clear the cloudy Front of wrinkled Care,*
> *And dry the tearful Sluices of Deſpair.*
> *Charm'd with that virtuous Draught, th' exalted Mind*
> *All Senſe of Woe delivers to the Wind*
> *Tho' on the blazing Pile his Parent lay,*
> *Or a lov'd Brother groan'd his Life away,*
> *Or darling Son oppreſſed by Ruffian-Force*
> *Fell breathleſs at his Feet, a mangled Corſe,*
> *From Morn to Eve, impaſſive and ſerene,*
> *The Man entranc'd would view the deathful Scene.*

In order to account in ſome Degree for theſe Effects mechanically, Mr COWPER examined a Solution of *Opium* with the Microſcope, and found its diſſolved Particles in the Shape of fringed Globules Whence he concludes, that ſuch Particles circulating in the Maſs of Blood, may be ſo intangled in its Serum, or thicken it in ſuch a manner, as to retard its Velocity when over-violent, and render its Motion calm and equal, whereby all painful Senſations will be taken off And from the ſame Principles it is eaſy to deduce all its other Effects, and become ſenſible how too great a Number of ſuch fringed Globules muſt cauſe a total Stagnation of the Blood, and conſequently kill —*Vid. Phil Tranſ* N° 222

An EXPLANATION of the SIXTEENTH PLATE.

The Seeds of Purſlain.

THE beauteous and orderly Configuration of theſe little Seeds makes them a very pleaſant Object for the Microſcope. They reſemble a good deal in Shape the Seed Nautilus or Sailor-Shell, being curled round in the Manner of a Spiral, at the larger End whereof, which repreſents the Mouth or Opening of the Shell, there appears a ſmall white tranſparent Subſtance, like a Skin, as repreſented by B B B B B The whole Surface is covered over with Abundance of little Protuberances, very regularly diſpoſed in ſpiral Rows, each of which ſeems nearly to reſemble the Wart on a Man's Hand The Inſide, when cut open, appears filled with a whitiſh-green pulpy Subſtance

There are divers Kinds of Seeds which imitate the Shape of much larger Bodies The Seed of *Scurvy-Graſs* nearly reſembles the Form of a *Concha Venerea*, or ſort of *Porcelain Shell* Thoſe of *Sweet-Marjoram* and *Pot-Marjoram* repreſent Olives. *Carrot-Seeds* are like the Cleft of a Cocoa Nut Huſk. The Seeds of *Succory* like a Quiver full of Arrows. Thoſe of the *Amaranthus* are delicately formed, ſomething like the Eye, and the black ſhrivell'd Seeds of *Onions* and *Leeks* are granulated all over in the manner of a Seal-ſkin The Mention of theſe is ſufficient to excite Curioſity to examine further, and a little Examination will diſcover numberleſs more Reſemblances

It is wonderful to obſerve by what various Means Providence guards and ſecures the Seeds of Vegetables from Danger and Deſtruction, in order to propagate, and, as it were, eternize every individual Species Some, as the Kernels of Apples and Pears, are placed in the Middle of a large Pulp, whoſe Subſtance both infolds and nouriſhes them Others, beſides the ſurrounding Pulp, are incloſed in thick Shells of Wood, as Plumbs, Peach, Nectarines, Apricocks, &c. Walnuts are guarded with a bitter Rind as well as a woody Shell, and Almonds, Cheſnuts, &c have a Covering armed with ſharp Prickles, to preſerve them from Injury till they arrive at Maturity Peaſe, Pears, Lentils, &c grow in Pods. The Seeds of Mulberries, Raſpberries, &c are placed in the little pulpy Grains of their Berries, and amongſt the moſt minute Seeds, ſome are covered with a Skin, others with a kind of Shell, and others ſtill with both

i N°-

Notwithſtanding the extreme Minuteneſs of many Kinds of Seeds, ſuch as *Fern, Harts-Tongue, Maiden-Hair*, and particularly of the *Puff-Ball*, which growing within it, ſeems, when the Ball is cruſhed, only like a Smoke or Vapour, but examined by the Microſcope, appears to be an infinite Number of Globules, whoſe Axis is not above the fiftieth Part of the Diameter of an Hair. So that a Cube of an Hair's-Breadth in Diameter, would be equal to an hundred and twenty five thouſand of them, each with a little Stalk or Tail. I ſay, notwithſtanding this extreme Minuteneſs, it is thought not an unreaſonable Suppoſition, that a little *Plantula*, or all the Parts of a perfect Plant, are folded together and included in every one of theſe little Grains, where, on being diſpoſed in Earth, or ſome other proper Bed, the Parts become unfolded and expanded, gradually, by a ſlow and progreſſive Inſinuation of Fluids adapted to the Diameters of their Veſſels, until, being ſtretched to the Bounds allotted them by Providence at their Formation, they reach their State of Perfection, or, in other Words, arrive at their full Growth.

MALPIGHI, LEEUWENHOEK, GREW, and ſeveral others, have diſcovered minute Plants, not only in the larger Seeds, ſuch as the Walnut, Cheſnut, Acorn, Beech-Nut, Seed of the Lime, Cotton-Seeds, &c. but alſo in the ſmaller of Radiſh, Hemp, Chervil, Scurvy-Graſs, Muſtard, &c. And we find in the *Philoſophical Tranſactions*, N° 457, an Account delivered to the *Royal Society*, by Mr. HENRY BAKER, Fellow of the ſaid Society, of a perfect Plant, found by Diſſection, in a Seed of the *Gramen tremulum*, with its Root and two Branches iſſuing from it, each of them producing ſeveral Leaves or Blades of Graſs. All which he preſented in a Slider, to be preſerved in the *Society*'s Repoſitory, together with a Drawing of them, which is printed in the ſaid *Tranſaction*. As therefore we have Demonſtration that ſuch minute Plants are to be found in many Seeds, we may reaſonably believe they really exiſt in all, however they may be concealed from our View, either by their Smalneſs, or the Manner of their fine Branchings or Ramifications amongſt the farinaceous or woody Parts of the Seed, which perhaps we never can develop, for Nature is uniform in all her Works, and ſeldom or never deviates from her general Plan.

Mr. BAKER juſt now mentioned, in a *Poem* of his called the UNIVERSE, publiſhed ſome Years ago, has ſome Lines ſo pertinent to this Subject, that we ſhall take the Liberty to ſubjoin them here.

> *Each Seed includes a Plant · that Plant, again,*
> *Has other Seeds, which other Plants contain.*
> *Thoſe other Plants have all their Seeds, and, Thoſe,*
> *More Plants, again, ſucceſſively, incloſe*
> *   Thus, every ſingle Berry that we find,*
> *Has, really, in itſelf whole Foreſts of its Kind*
> *Empire and Wealth one Acorn may diſpenſe,*
> *By Fleets to ſail a thouſand Ages hence.*
> *Each Myrtle-Seed includes a thouſand Groves,*
> *Where future Bards may warble forth their Loves.*
> *So ADAM's Loins contain'd his large Poſterity,*
> *All People that have been, and all that e'er ſhall be*
> *   Amazing Thought! what Mortal can conceive*
> *Such wond'rous Smalneſs!----Yet, we muſt believe*
> *What Reaſon tells : for Reaſon's piercing Eye*
> *Diſcerns thoſe Truths our Senſes can't deſcry*

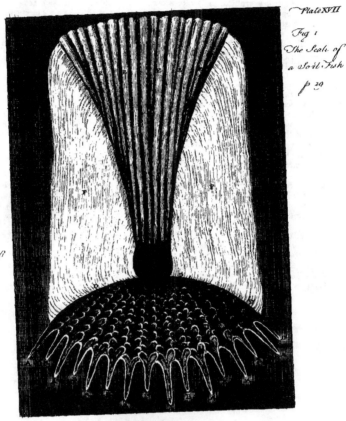

Plate XVII

Fig 1
The Scale of
a Soal Fish
p 29

Your James
the
Natural Bigness
p 29

Fig 2

a Piece of the Skin of a
Soal Fish with the Scales
sticking therein p 29

An EXPLANATION of the SEVENTEENTH PLATE.

FIG. 1.

The Scale of a Soal.

ON drawing the Finger along the Skin of a Soal, from the Tail upwards, we shall feel a Roughness that somewhat resists its Motion, the Cause of which will be explained by the Object now before us

This Figure represents the Scale of a Soal, plucked from the Skin, and viewed through a pretty large Magnifier. Its Shape is a Sort of oblong Square, that End within the Skin terminating circularly, and the other which comes out being armed with several sharp Prickles; every other of which A A A A is much longer than the intermediate ones B B B B

These Prickles are strong and sharp, and of a transparent Substance, having waved and indented Ridges running from them, with Furrows or Channels between those Ridges, appearing extremely pretty The two outermost Prickles on either Side, c c, extend wider than the Scale, and the semicircular Line, from their Points round by the Letters D, D, D, describes all that Part of it which rises out of the Skin, the other and much greater Part sticking fast and being buried in it. The Number of Prickles differs according to the Place whence the Scale is taken

From the Middle of the Part above described, to the End of the Part within the Skin, are a Number of small Quills or Pipes, E E E E, which probably convey Nourishment to the whole. These diminish gradually in Length on either side towards the Extremity, but spread, in Width, and form thereby a kind of fan-like Figure, which seems as it were fluted.

The two Sides F F, consist of a more fibrous Texture, having numberless little Ridges and Furrows, alternately, running parallel to each other, in a Curve-Direction at either End, though nearly strait about the Middle. The whole Scale appears grisly and transparent, but more particularly so in the little Channels between the Ridges: and all the Scales are pretty much like this, but not exactly so, for those growing on different Parts of the Fish differ from one another as well in Size as in many other Particulars unnecessary to mention here. G shews this same Scale about four times its natural Bigness

PLATE XVII. FIG. 2.

A Piece of the Skin of a Soal.

THE Skin being flead off from a pretty large Soal, and afterwards expanded and dried, the Inside thereof appeared to the naked Eye very like a Piece of Canvas, but the Microscope discovered that seeming Texture to be nothing else but the inner Ends of those curiously scallop'd Scales, which have been just now described in the former Figure. that is, the Ends of the Scales about E E E E were plainly visible by that Instrument, on the Back-side of the Skin, lying over one another like the Tiles upon a House.

The Outside of the Skin presented nothing more to the naked Eye than the usual Manner of arranging the Scales in a triangular Order, but seen through a Microscope, it exhibited a most curious and surprising Appearance, the Scales A A A A, being deeply fastened in the Skin B B, as the Figure before us shews

As no Object is more common than the Scale of a Soal amongst those prepared in Sliders, and sold by the People that make Microscopes, it is known almost by every Body, and the sharp prickly End is almost as generally imagined to be what sticks within the Skin, and the other what comes out of it; the quite contrary to which is here demonstrated to be true

The Skin and Scales on the Belly of a Soal are white, but on its Back of a greyish or Lead-Colour. The general Structure of the Scale is, however, the same on both Back and Belly, tho' there are particular Differences needless to be mentioned here, but the lead-colour'd ones on the Back are speckled very prettily with great Numbers of black minute Specks

The Scale of a Perch, tho' of a different Figure, has a Number of sharp Prickles standing out like those on the Soal's Scale

There is almost an infinite Variety in the Scales of Fishes, which seem analogous to the Feathers of Birds, and can't fail to afford Abundance of Entertainment and Satisfaction to those who will take the Pains attentively to examine them

I

An

An EXPLANATION of the EIGHTEENTH PLATE.

FIG. 1.

Couhage, or Cow-Itch.

Cow Itch   THE *Phafiolus filiqua hirfuta*, or *Hairy Kidney-Bean*, called in the *Eaſt-Indies* where it grows *Couhage*, is a Plant producing Pods like the common *French* Bean, but cluſter'd more together, and covered all over with ſhort brown Hairs, ſome of which being rubbed on the Back of one's Hand, or any other tender Part, cauſe a kind of painful Itching, troubleſome for a Time, but going off without any farther Miſchief. Theſe Hairs, wherewith waggiſh People divert themſelves ſometimes at the Expence of their Companions, by ſtrewing them on their Shirts or between their Sheets, are by Corruption uſually called *Cow-Itch*.

One of theſe Pods, about three Inches long, having ſix Beans in it, Dr HOOKE ſays was given him by a Sea-Captain. The whole Surface thereof was covered over with a thick and ſhining brown Down or Hair, which was very fine, and ſtiff for its Size. Rubbing ſome of this Down on the Back of his Hand, he found little or no Trouble therefrom at firſt, though he was ſenſible many of the ſharp Points were made to penetrate pretty deeply into the Skin, which made him doubtful whether it was the true *Couhage*. But ſoon after his Hand began to itch, and ſmarted in ſome Places, as if ſtung with a Flea or Gnat. This continued a pretty while, and by Degrees the Skin ſwelled with little red Puſtules; but enduring it without either ſcratching or rubbing, the Pain abated gradually, and was quite gone within an Hour, as were likewiſe the little Puſtules.

He then examined this Down by his Microſcope, and found it to be a Multitude of ſmall ſlender Bodies much reſembling Needles, ſuch as are repreſented by A B, C D, E F. They appeared very tranſparent, and ſeemed to be not hollow, tho' of that the Doctor could not be quite certain. Their Extremities A A A were very ſharp, ſtiff and hard, like the Subſtance of ſome Kinds of Thorns, and therefore being exceedingly minute they muſt eaſily by rubbing be thruſt into the tender Parts of the Skin, and occaſion quick and pungent, though not a violent Pain, which is the very Senſation we call Itching, and what even Horſe-Hairs ſhred ſmall, and ſtrewed between the Sheets will produce.

There may probably be more than one Sort of the *Couhage*, or perhaps the *Doctor* did not examine his with any conſiderable Magnifier: for having ſome of it at this preſent time under one of the greateſt Magnifiers, in order to give a juſt Deſcription thereof, (which is the Method taken as often as the Objects can be got, to render theſe Accounts exactly agreeable to Truth) there are many minute *Spiculæ* plainly to be diſcerned on every Side of the little Hairs, pointing backwards like the Beards of a Javelin, by which Conformation when once they enter they cannot eaſily be withdrawn.

We have in our own Gardens ſome Species of the *Phaſioli*, the Pods whereof are covered like the *Couhage* with brown Hairs, which if rubbed on the Skin, when the Pods are full ripe, and the Hairs themſelves grown ſtiff and hard by being dry, produce nearly the ſame Effects, though when green and moiſt they are ſoft and pliable, and entirely harmleſs. Of this Nature are the *Lupines*, yellow, blue, and white, and likewiſe the *ſweet-ſcented* or *perfumed Peaſe*.

PLATE XVIII. FIG. 2.

The Sting of a Bee.

   A Bee's Sting, the Doctor tells us, appears through the Microſcope to be a Sheath without a Chape or Top, in Form like the Holſter of a Piſtol, beginning at *d*, and ending at *b*, which Sheath he plainly diſtinguiſhed to be hollow, containing a Sword or Dart within it, together with a poiſonous Liquor, which being conveyed into the Wound it makes, occaſions a moſt ſevere Pain.

This Sheath or Caſe appeared to have ſeveral Joinings marked 1, 2, 3, 4, 5, 6, 7, and was armed near the Top on both ſides with ſeveral ſharp tranſparent Thorns, Hooks or Points, growing out of little Protuberancies, as repreſented *p p*, *q q*, *r r*, *s s*, *t t*, *v v*. Which Hooks the Creature ſpreads out, or draws in, occaſionally, as a Cat does her Claws.

The Sword or Dart which is lodged within the Sheath, appeared as in the Figure, with its ſharp End *a b* protruded beyond the ſaid Sheath like a Sword in a Scabbard

1   without

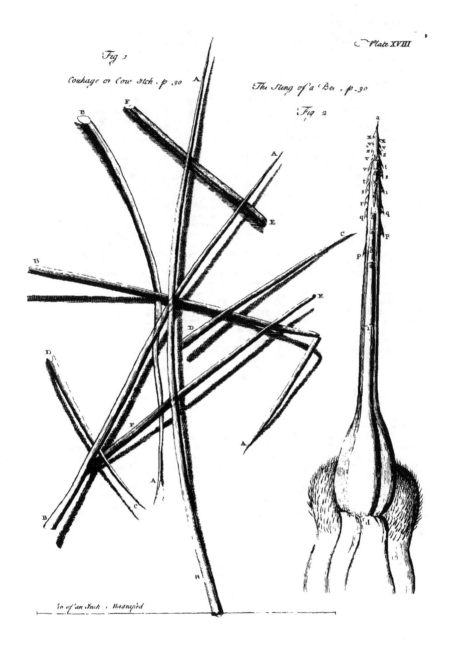

Plate XVIII

Fig 1

Couhage or Cow Itch. p.30

The Sting of a Bee. p.30

Fig 2

¼ of an Inch Magnified

without a Chape. This Point was likewise armed on both fides with Thorns or Hooks, *x x*, *y y*, *z z*, exactly like thofe before defcribed, which can alfo be extended or pulled in juft as the Creature pleafes

Such a Structure fhews the Ufe of the Hooks to be very confiderable towards thruft-ing in the Sting as well as fixing it For the Point, which is extremely fharp, being thruft eafily into the Skin of any Animal, the Bee (when once 'tis entered) by endeavour-ing to pull it back into the Sheath (whilft its Hooks on either Side lay faft hold on the Skin) draws the Top of the Sheath into the Skin after it, and then the fixing of the Hooks on both Sides the Sheath, *p p*, *q q*, *r r*, &c into the Skin, not only keeps the Sheath from fliding back, but furthers its Paffage inwards, and thus, by an alternate and fuccef-five retracting and emitting of the Sting in and out of the Sheath, the little angry Creature can penetrate by Degrees even the tough Hide of a Bear, one of its moft deadly Enemies This Sort of Motion to and fro, does alfo perhaps pump up the poifonous Juice, and make it hang in a Drop at the End of the Sheath *b* And thefe Hooks are probably the Reafon why a Bee, when haftily driven away upon ftinging, frequently leaves its Weapon fticking in the Flefh, thereby caufing the painful Symptoms to be greater and more laft-ing.

We fee here the Subftance of what Dr *Hooke* fays concerning a Bee's Sting, but later Obfervers have found fome Miftakes in his Account, for no Beards are really to be difco-vered on the Sheath or Cafe, which on the contrary is perfectly fmooth and polifhed, neither has it any Joints, or is parted in two, as his Figure makes it, nor does it termi-nate in a bluntifh Point, but a very fharp one: Neither is the bearded Weapon always fticking out beyond the Sheath, as he reprefents it, nor indeed does it ever come out at the very Extremity, but at an Orifice below it, and that only in the Act of ftinging This Part alfo is greatly mifreprefented, for a Couple of *bearded Spears* or *Darts* are included within the Sheath, whereas he fuppofes no more than one, the Beards too are placed only on one Side of each Dart, and not all round them But as a full and true Defcription may be defired by fome Readers, 'tis hoped what follows, taken from the *Microfcope made eafy*, will not be thought fuperfluous

" The Sting of a Bee is a horny Sheath or Scabbard that includes two bearded Darts.
" This Sheath ends in a fharp Point, near the Extremity whereof a Slit opens, through
" which, at the Time of Stinging, *two bearded Darts* are protruded beyond the End of
" the Sheath, one whereof being a little longer than the other, fixes its Beard firft, but
" the other inftantly following, they penetrate alternately, deeper and deeper, taking hold
" of the Flefh with their Hooks, till the whole Sting becomes buried in the Wound,
" and then a venomous Juice is injected through the fame Sheath, from a little Bag at
" the Root of the Sting, which occafions an acute Pain, and a fwelling of the Part,
" continuing fometimes feveral Days. This is beft prevented by enlarging the Wound
" immediately to give it fome Difcharge."

" Mr. *Derham* fays, he counted in the Sting of a Wafp, eight Beards on the Side
" of each Dart, fomewhat like the Beards of Fifh-Hooks, and the fame Number has been
" obferved in that of a Bee. When thefe Beards are ftruck deep in the Flefh, if the
" wounded Perfon ftarts before the Bee can difengage them, fhe leaves her Sting behind,
" fticking in the Wound · But if he has Patience to ftand quiet till fhe brings the Hooks
" clofe down to the Side of the Darts, fhe withdraws her Weapon, and the Wound
" becomes much lefs painful.

" To view the Sting of a Bee by the Microfcope, cut off the End of its Tail, and
" then touching it with a Pin or Needle, it will thruft out the Sting and Darts, which
" may be fnipt off with a Pair of Sciffars for Obfervation. Alfo, if you catch a Bee in
" a Leather Glove, its Sting will be left therein, being unable to difengage its Hooks
" from Leather : And when it is quite dead, which it will not be till after feveral Hours,
" you may by Care and Gentlenefs extract it with its Darts and Hooks By fqueezing
" the Tail, pulling out the Sting, and preffing it at the Bottom, you may likewife force
" up the Darts : But without fome Practice this will be a little difficult "

The Bag containing the poifonous Juice may eafily be found at the Bottom of the Sting, being commonly pulled out with it.

An EXPLANATION of the NINETEENTH PLATE.

The Figures in this Plate ſhew the Conſtruction of the Feathers of Birds.

FIG. 1.

A minute Part of a Gooſe's Feather.

A Goofe's
Feather

A Middle-ſized Gooſe-Quill being examined by the naked Eye, it was eaſy enough to diſtinguiſh, that the main Stem ſent forth on either ſide about three hundred little *Arms*. Thoſe on the one ſide being longer and more downy, thoſe on the other much more ſtiff and ſhort. Many of the downy longer *Arms* being viewed with an ordinary Microſcope, were found each of them to have along one of its upper Edges near twelve hundred ſmall *Branches*, (if we may ſo call them) ſuch as E F, and on its other Edge, the ſame Number as L, I.

'Tis here proper to take notice, that each of the little *Arms* is of a tapering Shape from its iſſuing out of the Stem to its Extremity, where it ends in a fine Point, that it is not a round Body, but reſembles the Half of a long Cone, being concave on one ſide, and on the other convex, its Breadth making an acute Angle with the Length of the Stem · That the middle or moſt convex Part is fine and membranous, its Under-Edge being an extremely ſmooth and thin *Film*, but the *upper* and *outer Edge* ends flat, and thereby forms two other *hairy Edges*, each having a different Sort of *Hairs*, laminated, or ſomewhat broad at Bottom, but ſlender and bearded upwards ---*Note*, The Concavity of the Arms makes them readily fall into one another

The flat upper Edge, and the two Edges made thereby, are ſhewn by a tranſverſe Section I N O E, and the two Kinds of *Hairs* or little *Branches* by E F, L I.

Each of the *Branches* E F ſeemed to have ſixteen or eighteen Joints, out of which ſmall long *Fibres* or *Tendrils* iſſued, gradually longer or ſhorter than one another, according to their Poſition along the Branch E F, thoſe on the Under-ſide, *viz* 1, 2, 3, 4, 5, 6, 7, 8, 9, &c. being much longer than thoſe directly againſt them on the Upper, and ſeveral of them as 3, 4, 5, 6, 7, 8, 9, were terminated with ſuch ſmall Hooks, as are viſible to the naked Eye on the Seed-Buttons of the Bur-dock.

The Fibres on the other Edge L I appeared to have near as many knotted Joints, but without any Tendrils or Hooks, each of them about the Middle K ſeeming to divide into a Kind of Fork, one Part whereof, namely K L, was nearly the ſame Length as K I, the other M was very ſhort.

PLATE XIX. FIG. 2.

Two Parts of a Gooſe's Quill.

THE wonderful Structure of the Parts juſt now deſcribed, deſerves the moſt ſerious Attention and Conſideration as to their Uſe In order to explain which the more readily, the Figure under our Eye was given

We ſee here two Pieces of the downy Arms I N, E O, placed, as to one another, in the ſame manner as they appear upon the Quill, at the Diſtance of I F, or ſomewhat more. The collateral Branches *a a a a*, *b b b b*, are ſo ranged that they lie upon and croſs over one another, by which means the hooked Ends of the Tendrils on the Branches of one Arm, getting between the naked Branches of the Arm next to them, which are full of Knots, the Hooks of the Tendrils claſp round thoſe Knots, and faſten all the Parts ſo cloſely and admirably together, as to hinder even the Air from paſſing through them. And though the Thickneſs of one of theſe Tendrils amounts not to the five hundredth Part of an Inch, they all together form ſo ſtrong a Texture, that the exceeding quick and violent beating of them againſt the Air by the Strength of the Bird's Wing, is unable to diſjoin them.

The Contrivance and Fabrick of the numberleſs little Parts which conſtitute a Feather, taken either ſeparately or together, ſtrongly prove the Wiſdom of Providence, and its Care of all its Creatures, even in the minuteſt Matters, for their Contexture is ſuch, that if the component Parts ſhould be violently diſjoined by any external Injury, (ſeveral of which Separations would prevent the Bird from flying) they for the moſt part, by a
kind

2

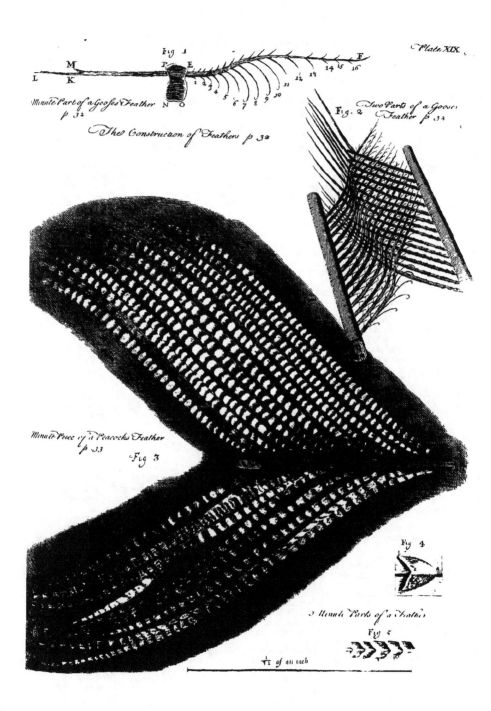

Plate XIX.

Fig. 1

M

L K

P E

N O

F

14 15 16

1 2 3 4 5 6 7 8 9 10 11 12 13

Minute Part of a Goofes Feather
p 32

The Construction of Feathers p 32

Fig. 2 Two Parts of a Goose
Feather p 32

Minute Piece of a Peacocks Feather
p 33

Fig 3

Fig 4

3 Minute Parts of a Feather

Fig 5

1/12 of an inch

kind of Springinefs or Elafticity readily come together of themfelves, and re-unite Or elfe by the Birds ftroaking the Feather, or drawing it through its Bill, they all become fettled and woven into their former and natural Pofture. In fhort, there are fuch an infinite Company of hooked Tendrils ready to catch hold of the jointed Fibres, that they muft necefiarily hang together whenever they come to meet, and though the Square Holes, which they form by crofling over one another, and which are vifibly open and pervious, appear by the Microfcope to be more than half the Surface of the Feather, it feems reafonable to believe, however extraordinary, that the Air does not pafs through them.

PLATE XIX. FIG 3, 4, 5.

Parts of a Peacock's Feather.

'TIS plain, by the naked Eye, that the Stem of each Feather in the Tail of a Peacock, fends out Multitudes of *lateral Branches*, and that each of thefe *lateral Branches* has innumerable little *Sprigs, Threads* or *Hairs*, iffuing on either Side of it, from End to End. A Peacock's Feather

The Figure before us fhews about the thirty-fecond Part of an Inch in Length of one of thefe *lateral Branches*, as examined by the Microfcope

A, B Point out the middle or ftem-like Part cut off at both Ends.

CD, CD, CD, Reprefent the *Hairs* or *Threads* iffuing therefrom, each of which appears to be a long Body, of fome Breadth, with a Multitude of bright reflecting Parts, whofe Form and Shape cannot eafily be determin'd, fince they change continually, and feem very different in different Pofitions to the Light. nay, only interpofing one's Hand between them and the Light, or even putting up or pulling down a Safh very much changes their Appearance However, by frequent Examinations, compared with one another, 'tis hoped the true Figure is here determin'd.

Thefe Threads are found, therefore, to confift of Rows of fmall *Laminæ* or *Plates*, fuch as EEEE. each of which is fhaped much like *Fig.* 4, *a b c d*. where the Part *a c* being a Ridge or little Stem, and *b, d*, the Corners of two fmall thin Plates growing from the faid Stem in the Middle, make together a Kind of little Feather Thefe little Plates or Feathers lie clofe to, and partly over one another, like a Number of floping ridge or gutter Tyles They grow oppofite to one another, on each Side of the Stem, by two and two, from Bottom to Top; the Tops of the lower covering the Roots of the next above them, in the Manner reprefented *Fig.* 5

Each of thefe laminated Bodies is on the under Side of a very opake Subftance, that fufiers very few Rays to be reflected, but their upper Sides, confifting of exceeding thin Plates, lying clofe together, do thereby, like Mother of Pearl, not only reflect a very bright Light, but tinge that Light in a moft curious Manner, and, by means of various Pofitions in refpect of the Light, they reflect back now one Colour, and then another, and that moft vividly And hence we may account for all the gaudy and beauteous Colours which adorn the Feathers of this and many other Birds Namely, from the exceeding Smallnefs and Finenefs of the reflecting Parts.

K An

An EXPLANATION of the TWENTIETH PLATE.

FIG. 1.

The Foot of a Fly.

A Fly's Foot   THE Foot of a Fly is the Object now before us, confisting of three Joints, two Talons, and as many Pattens, Soles, or Spunges, as they are called by some. By the wonderful Contrivance of which Instruments this Creature is enabled to walk perpendicularly upwards, even against the Sides of Glafs; nay to fufpend itfelf, and walk with its Body downwards, on the Ceilings of Rooms, and the under Surfaces of most other Things, with as much feeming Facility and Firmnefs, as if it were a kind of *Antipode*, and had a Tendency upwards. but the quite contrary is evident from its being unable to fufpend itfelf on the under Surface of a clean and well-polifh'd Glafs

The two Talons are handfomely fhaped, in the Manner reprefented A B, and A C, and are very large in Proportion to the reft of the Foot. The bigger Part of them from A to *d d*, is briftled or hairy all over, but from thence towards C and B, the Tops or Points which turn downwards and inwards, are fmooth and very fharp. Each Talon moves on a Joint at A, whereby the Fly is able to fhut or open them at Pleafure: So that the Points B, and C, having enter'd the Pores of any Thing, and the Fly endeavouring to fhut its Talons, they not only draw againft, and by that means faften each other, but alfo pull forwards all the Parts of the Foot G G, A, D D: and at the fame Time the Tenters or fharp Points G G G G (whereof a Fly has two at every Joint) run into the Pores, if they find any, or, on a foft Place, make their own Way.

Somewhat of this Kind may be difcerned by the naked Eye in the Feet of a *Chafer*, and if it be fuffered to creep over the Hand or any tender Part of the Body, its Manner of Stepping will be as fenfible to the Feeling as to the Sight.

But as the *Chafer*, notwithftanding this Contrivance to faften its Claws, often falls when it attempts to walk on hard and clofe Bodies, fo likewife would the Fly, had not Nature furnifh'd his Foot with a couple of Pattens or Spunges D D, which we are now going to defcribe

From the Bottom or under Part of the laft Joynt of the Foot K, two fmall thin plated horny Subftances proceed, each confifting of two flat Pieces D D Thefe, about F F, *f f*, feem to be flexible like the Covers of a Book, whereby the two Sides *e e, e e*, do not always lie in the fame Plane, but may fometimes fhut clofer, fo that each of them can take a little hold. But this is not all, for the Bottoms of thefe Spunges are every where befet with fmall Briftles or Tenters, like the Wire Teeth in a *Wool-Card*, with all their Points inclining forwards by which the two Talons drawing the Foot forwards, as before defcribed, and the Spunges being applyed to the Surface of the Body the Fly walks upon, with the Points of all their Briftles looking forwards and outwards, as expreffed in the Figure *o o o o*, if the Surface of the Body has any Irregularity, or gives Way in any Manner, the Fly can fufpend itfelf, or walk thereon very eafily and firmly. And its being able to walk on Glafs, proceeds partly from fome little Ruggednefs thereon, but chiefly from a Kind of Tarnifh or dirty fmoky Subftance, which adheres to the Surface of that very hard Body, fo that although the fharp Points on the Spunges cannot penetrate the Surface of Glafs, they may eafily enough catch hold of the Tarnifh it has contracted.

Some indeed have fuppofed thefe Spunges filled with an imaginary Glew, which fixes the Fly, in fuch a Manner as to prevent its falling, but if there was fuch a fticky Matter, 'tis not eafy to conceive how the Feet could fo readily again be loofen'd, and and move fo nimbly forwards. And as our Senfes can furnifh us with a rational Way of performing this by the curious Mechanifm of the Parts employ'd, 'twould be wrong to introduce unintelligible Explications

y y y are fome very long, ftiff, fharp-pointed Hairs or Briftles

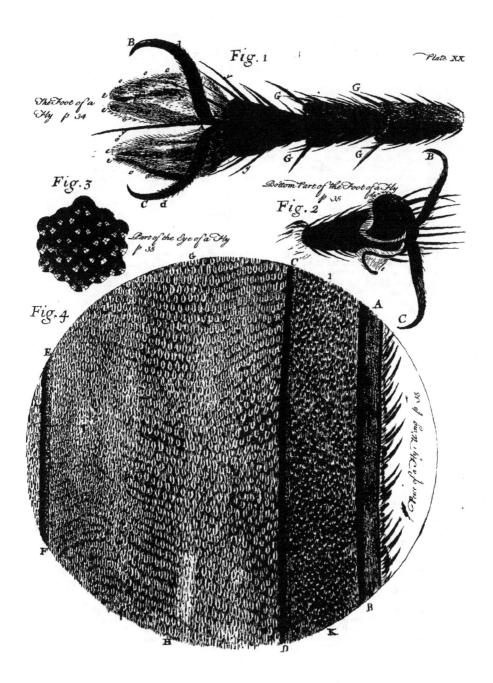

Fig. 1

The Foot of a
Fly p 34

Plate. XX

Fig. 3

Fig. 2

Bottom Part of the Foot of a Fly
p 35

Part of the Eye of a Fly
p 35

Fig. 4

PLATE XX. FIG. 2.

Another Foot of a Fly.

THIS fhews us only the Bottom Joint of the Foot, with the Talons having their hooked Point B C extended, and the Spunges *d e* bending inwards, in order to take hold of any Thing We fee alfo more plainly in this Figure the Joints whereby the Talons perform their Motions. A Fly's Foot

The Foot is likewife fhaded with a Growth of Hairs, which like a Biufh ferves to clean the Fly's Wings and Eyes, an Office fhe employs it in very frequently. And indeed it is a pretty Amufement to fee her perform this Exercife, for firft fhe cleans her Brufhes, by rubbing her Paws one againft another, then draws them over her Wings, and afterwards under them, and at laft concludes with brufhing her Eyes and Head: by which means fhe cleans away all little Particles of Duft or Smoke, that may cloud her Eyes, or fettle on her Wings

PLATE XX. FIG. 3.

Part of a Fly's Eye.

THIS little Piece of the pearled Eye of a Fly, confifting of nineteen Pearls or Hemifpheres (a particular Defcription whereof will be given in the next Plate) is here introduced, as it appeared before the Microfcope, to fhew how perfectly the Images of Objects are reflected from their fmooth and polifhed Surfaces, infomuch that Houfes, Trees, and Landfcapes of every Thing within a certain Diftance, may be difcovered on them, in the fame manner as on the fmall Balls of Quickfilver, but not near fo lively. The Reflection from thefe being fomewhat languid, as it is from Water, Glafs, Chryftal, and fuch-like Bodies Pea of a Fly's Eye

The Image of two Windows in the Chamber where they were examined, is expreffed on each of thefe. More will be faid in the next Plate concerning the Eyes of Infects.

PLATE XX. FIG. 2.

Part of a Fly's Wing.

A Whole Wing (of which this is only a Part) is exhibited *Plate* XXII *Fig* 2. to exprefs its Form in general But the Piece here before us is magnified a great deal more, to afford a clearer Notion of its wonderful Structure and Materials. Part of a Fly's Wing

It confifts plainly of a fine thin tranfparent Skin or Membrane, varioufly folded, platted and diftended over the whole Area, and feveral Bones, Ribs, or Stems, difpofed with great Regularity and Contrivance, fo as to ftrengthen and fupport the Wing, and determine its proper Figure

A B, C D, E F, are the Bones or Ribs of the Wing, each of which is manifeftly covered with Multitudes of little Scales, and A B, in particular, which is the largeft Bone of the whole Wing, and may properly enough be called the *Cut-Air*, being that which terminates and ftiffens the foremoft Edge of the Wing, is not only covered with Scales lying regularly one over another, but its Fore-Edge is armed with great Numbers of little Briftles, all the Points of which are directed towards the Tip of the Wing · And even the whole Edge all round the Wing is covered with a fmall Fringe, confifting of fhorter and more flender Briftles

G H, I K, The fine Membrane extended between thefe bony Ribs, if examined by the firft or fecond Magnifier, and in a clean and proper Light, will be feen thickly ftuck with innumerable minute fharp-pointed Hairs or Briftles, ranged in the moft regular Rows, over its whole Surface, and intermingled with thefe may be perceived a like Number of little Pits or black Spots, which feem to be the Roots of the Hairs growing on the other Side.

In feveral other Flies, there are infinite Numbers of fmall Fibres which cover both Sides of this thin Membrane, inftead of minute Hairs. And on moft Moths and Butterflies, they don't only refemble the Feathers of Birds in the Manner of their Arrangement, but are variegated with the fame kind of curious and lively Colours which the Feathers of Birds exhibit

2   An

An EXPLANATION of the TWENTY-FIRST PLATE.

The Eye and Head of a Drone-Fly.

Face and
Eyes of a
Drone

THE Object we are going to describe is the Face-Part (if it may be called so) and Eyes of a grey *Drone-Fly*, whose Head being cut off, and fixed with the Face or Fore-part upwards, before the Microscope, appeared as in the Figure under our View at present.

This Insect is remarkable for having a larger Head in proportion to its Body, and bigger Clusters of Eyes in proportion to its Head, than any of the small Flies. It has also a greater Variety in the Balls or Pearls of each Cluster than Flies commonly have, and therefore was thought the properest Subject for Examination as to the Eyes of such-like Creatures

The greatest Part of the Head consisted of two large semicircular and regular Protuberances or Eyes, A B C D E, the Surfaces of which were covered all over with, or shaped into Multitudes of minute Hemispheres, disposed in a triagonal Order, and in that Order forming exact and equidistant Rows, with little Trenches or Furrows between each

These Hemispheres were of different Sizes in different Parts of each Eye, the lowermost Half of them looking downwards, *viz* C D E, C D E, being a great deal smaller than the Half A B C E, A B C E, looking upwards, fore-right, sideways and backwards; a Variety unobserved in any other small Fly

Every one of these Hemispheres seemed very near the true and exact Shape of an half Globe, with a Surface exceeding smooth and regular, and reflected the Images of Objects, as described before, *Plate XX Fig* 3.

There were fourteen thousand *Pearls* or *Hemispheres* distinguishable in the Clusters of this Fly, as was computed by numbering some Rows of them several Ways, and casting up the whole Amount, for each Cluster was thereby found to contain about seven thousand Pearls, *viz.* three thousand of the larger Size, and four thousand of the smaller, whose Rows were more thick and close.

Now that each of these *Pearls* or *Hemispheres* is a perfect Eye, there can be little reason to doubt, each being furnished with a *Cornea*, with a *transparent Humour*, and with an *Uvea* or *Retina*. The Figure of each is also very spherical, exactly polished, and exceeding lively and plump, when the Fly is living, as in greater Animals, and likewise, as in them, dull, shrunk, and flaccid, when the Fly is dead.

One of the Clusters being cut from the Head, and opened, a clear Liquor, tho' exceeding little in Quantity, was discovered by the Microscope, immediately under the outward Skin or Covering, which Covering seemed perfectly to resemble the *Cornea* of a Man's Eye, and when a darkish Matter that lay behind was removed, appeared transparent, with as many Cavities within-side, and ranged in the same Order as the little Hemispheres on its outer Surface

Thus, each of these Pearls or Hemispheres being covered with a transparent protuberant *Cornea*, and containing a Liquor correspondent to the watery or glassy Humours of the Eye, must necessarily refract all the parallel Rays falling on it, into a Point not far within, where probably the *Retina* is placed, which *Retina*, in all likelihood, is that dark opake Matter just now mentioned, appearing by the Microscope to be placed a little more than the Diameter of the Pearl below or within the *Tunica Cornea* And if so, there is in all probability a little Picture or Image of external Objects, painted at the Bottom, upon the *Retina* of every one of these Hemispheres to which such Objects happen to be opposite But, as in a Man's Eye, though a Picture or Sensation is impressed on the *Retina* of all the Objects lying almost in an Hemisphere, some very few Points only placed in, or near the *Optic Axis*, are discerned distinctly, so Multitudes of Pictures of an Object may be made in as many Pearls, and yet no distinct Vision be produced but in one, or some very few, that are directly, or almost directly opposite to the Object. And notwithstanding it has pleased God to give these Sorts of Creatures such Multitudes of Eyes, 'tis very likely their observing Faculty is employed only about some one Object, for which they have most Concern

The most remarkable of all the Insects we know for its fine pearled Eyes, is the *Libella* or *Dragon-Fly* Mr LEEUWENHOEK reckons twelve thousand five hundred forty four *Lenses* in each Eye of this Creature, or twenty five thousand eighty-eight in both, placed in an hexangular Position, each *Lens* having six others round it He observed likewise in the Center of each *Lens* a minute transparent Spot brighter than the rest, and

i   supposed

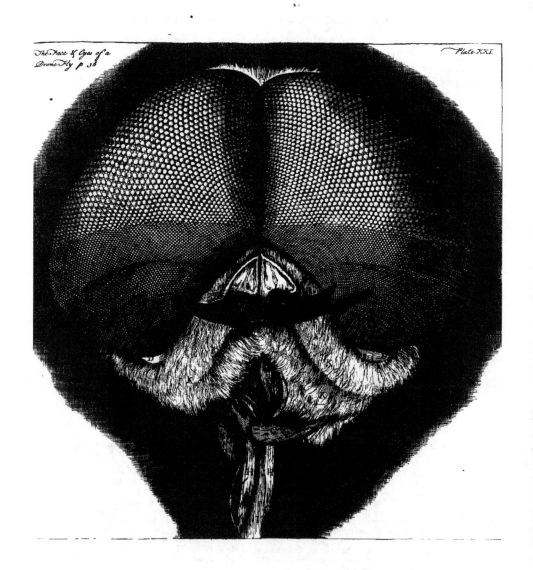

The Face & Eyes of a
Drone Fly p 36

Plate XXI

suppofed to be the *Pupil* through which the Rays of Light are tranfmitted upon the *Retina*. This Spot had three Circles furrounding it, and feemed feven Times lefs than the Diameter of the whole *Lens* He alfo numbered fix thoufand two hundred thirty-fix Pearls or Hemifpheres in a *Silkworm*'s two Eyes, when in the Fly State: three thoufand one hundred eighty-one in each Eye of a *Beetle*, and eight thoufand in the two Eyes of a *common Fly*.

    The Author of *Spectacle de la Nature* finely obferves, * that the Eyes of other Creatures are as it were multiplyed by Motion: whereas thofe of a Fly are fixed and immoveable, and can only fee what lies directly before them, they are very numerous therefore, and are placed in a round Surface, fome in a high, others in a low Situation, to inform the Fly of every Thing wherein fhe may be interefted. She has a Number of Enemies, but, with the Aid of thefe Eyes that furround her Head, fhe is enabled to difcover whatever Danger threatens from above, behind, or on either Side, even when fhe is in full Purfuit of a Prey directly before her.

    Thefe *Eyes* or little *Hemifpheres* are placed, in all Kinds of Flies and aerial Animals, in a moft neat, regular, and admirable Ordination of *triangular* Rows, ranged as near to one another as poffible, and leaving the leaft Pits or Furrows between them that can poffibly be. But in *Crabs, Lobfters, Shrimps*, and fuch Kinds of *cruftaceous Water Animals*, (whofe Eyes are lefs pearled,) the Pearls are ranged in a quadrangular Order, the Rows interfecting at right Angles, by which Difpofition their Number on equal Surfaces muft be lefs. but to make them a Recompence for this, kind Nature has formed their Eyes a little moveable, whereas thofe of flying Infects are all fixt

    The Goodnefs of Providence is particularly diftinguifhable in the Formation and Situation of the Eyes of different Animals, in a Manner moft fuitable to their different Necefities and Ways of Living In *Hares* and *Rabbets*, whofe Safety depends on flight, they are very protuberant, and placed fo much towards the Sides of their Head, that their two Eyes take in nearly a whole Sphere. whereas in *Dogs* (that purfue them) the Eyes are fet more forward in the Head, to look that Way more than backward.

    In *Cats* the Pupil being erect, and the fhutting of the Eye-Lids tranfverfe thereto, they can fo clofe the Pupil, as to admit, as it were, one only fingle Ray of Light: and, on the contrary, by throwing all open, they can take in all the fainteft Rays. Which is an incomparable Provifion for Animals that have Occafion to watch and way-lay their Prey both by Day and Night. But befides this, fome nocturnal Creatures have a certain Radiation or darting out of Rays of Light from their Eyes, enabling them to catch their Prey in the Dark: and this moft People have been Witneffes of in Cats.

    Notwithftanding Aristotle, Pliny, Albertus Magnus, and feveral other Writers were of Opinion that *Moles* are blind, the greater Diligence of the Moderns in Diffections and Experiments have found them to have Eyes moft excellently fitted for their fubterraneous Way of Life not indeed much bigger than a large Pin's Head, but which, it is fuppofed they have a Faculty of withdrawing, if not quite into the Head, yet more or lefs within the Hair, as they have more or lefs Occafion to employ or guard them †.

    The Eyes of *Snails* are placed at the Ends of their Horns, and are thruft out at fome Diftance, or drawn quite within the Head as the Animal thinks proper.

    Thofe of the *Camelion* turn backwards, or any Way elfe, like a Lens or convex Glafs in a verfatile globular Socket, without any Motion of the Head, ‡ and it is very extraordinary to fee one of the Eyes of this Creature moving, whilft the other remains fixt: one turning forwards at the fame Time the other looks behind, or perhaps one looking up to the Sky, when the other turns itfelf downwards towards the Ground

    Several Opinions have prevailed amongft the Anatomifts about the Reafon why Man having two Eyes fees not an Object double GALEN and his Difciples thought this to arife from a Coalition or Decuffation of the optic Nerves, but do not well agree whether they decuffate, coalefce or only touch one another. The Bartholines affert they are united, ‖ not fimply by Contact, or Interfection, but by a total Confufion or Commixture of their Subftance. Vesalius and fome others have found a few Inftances of their being difunited, but fay it is generally otherwife. Dr. Gibson tells us, § they are united by the clofeft Conjunction, but not Confufion of their Fibres. Des Cartes, and fome befides, judge this to be not from any Coalefcence, Contact, or croffing of the optic Nerves, but from a Sympathy between them. For, fays Des Cartes, the *Fibrillæ* conftituting the medullary Part of thofe Nerves being fpread in the *Retina* of each Eye,

* Dialogue viii   † Derham's Phyf Theol p 94   ‡ Vid Phil Tranf N° 137 Mem for a Nat Hift
of Anat at Par p 22   ‖ Bartholin Anat lib 3 c 2   § Gibfon's Anat lib 3 c 10

have

have each of them corresponding Parts in the Brain : so that when any of those *Fibrillæ* are struck by any Part of an Object, the corresponding Parts of the Brain are thereby affected, and the Soul thereby informed.   The Archbishop of *Cambray* says, we never see an Object double, because the two Nerves that are subservient to Sight in our Eyes, are but two Branches that unite in one Pipe, as the two Glasses of a Pair of Spectacles unite in the upper Part that joins them both together.   And lastly, our great Sir Isaac Newton, with his usual Modesty, hints to us his Opinion by the Way of Query.   Are not the Species of Objects (says he) seen with both Eyes, united where the optic Nerves meet, before they come into the Brain, the Fibres on the right Side of both Nerves uniting there &c? For the optic Nerves of such Animals as look the same Way with both Eyes (such as of Men, Dogs, Sheep, Oxen, &c) meet before they come into the Brain: but the optic Nerves of such Animals as do not look the same way with both Eyes, as of Fishes, and of the Camelion, do not meet, if I am rightly informed *.

After this Digression, which 'tis hoped may be excusable on so curious a Subject, we shall return to finish the Explanation of this Plate, wherein

F F shew the Horns.
G G the Smellers or Feelers.
H H and I the Proboscis.
K K K K the Hairs and Bristles

All which will be described in explaining the following Plate.

An EXPLANATION of the TWENTY-SECOND PLATE.

FIG. 1.

A Blue-Fly, or Flesh-Fly.

Blue-Bottle Fly

WE see here the *Blue-Bottle* or *common Flesh-Fly*, enlarged by the Microscope, in such a Manner, as to shew distinctly all its particular and minute Members and Ornaments.

A A, Its protuberant and pearled Eyes, which make a considerable Part of the Head, though much smaller than those of the *Drone-Fly*, described in the last Plate.   These Pearls or Hemispheres were ranged in the same triangular Order as in that Fly, but without any such Difference in Size.

B B, A scaly prominent Front between the Eyes, adorned and armed with large tapering sharp black Bristles, which growing on either Side in Rows, and bending towards each other near the Top, form a Kind of Arch of Bristles, that almost covers the Front B B.

C, a Projecting Part at the anterior End of this Arch, and about the Middle of the Face, on which grow D D, two little oblong Bodies, not unlike the *Apices* or *Pendants* in Lillies, each having one small Joint where it unites to C, and another that joins it to the Front Part B.----- These in the Head of the *Drone-Fly* are called Horns, from the great Resemblance they bear to the Horns of some Kinds of Beasts.

E E, Brushy Bristles or Feathers, somewhat like the Tufts of a *Cock-Gnat*, growing from the upper Part and Outsides of the Horns, D D

F F, Four strong Bristles, placed two and two, and bending towards each other, just above the Opening of the Mouth.

G H I, The Fly's *Proboscis* or *Trunk*, coming out from the Middle of the Mouth. It seems to be a hollow Body, and by means of several Joints is moved to and fro, thrust out or pulled in at pleasure.   There's a Knee or Bending expressed at H, which from thence to the Extremity is slit, as it were, into two Lips, H I, H I, which on their outer Sides are covered with pretty large Hairs, though the Hairs on the upper Part of the *Proboscis* are very small.   These Lips open or shut easily, and serve to hold or take in little Pieces of solid Food , but when the Fly sucks any thing from the Surface of a Body, she spreads them open, and applies their hollow Part perfectly close thereto , in which Condition they become a kind of Pump, to draw up the Juices of Fruits or other Liquors.

                                                                            K K,

* Newton's Opt. Q. 15

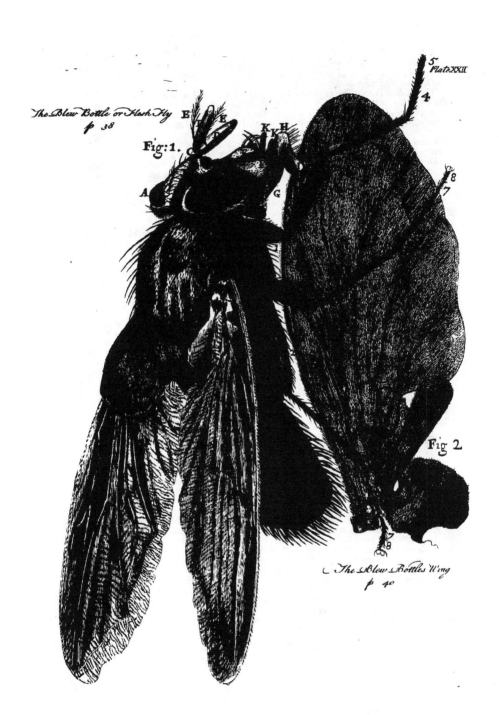

The Blew Bottle or Flesh Fly
p 38

Fig: 1.

Plate XXII

Fig 2

The Blew Bottles Wing
p 40

K K, Two little hairy oblong Bodies, growing within the Mouth from either Side of the *Proboscis*. These Parts are differently shaped, and much larger in the Head of the *Drone-Fly*, where they are marked G G. Dr. HOOKE imagines these may probably be its Organs of Smelling

The Middle-Part or *Thorax* of this Fly is crustaceous, and strongly made, rounded on the Top, and covered with large long black Bristles, standing like the Quills of a Porcupine, in parallel Order, all pointing towards the Tail. From the hinder and under Part grow out three large Legs on each Side, (as represented in the Figure) all covered with a strong hairy Shell, and resembling the Legs of a Crab or Lobster Each Leg is jointed, and made up of eight Parts, 1, 2, 3, 4, 5, 6, 7, 8; on the eighth of which grow the *Soles* or *Spunges*, and *Claws*, described before in the *Twentieth Plate*

Of these six Legs she seldom employs any more than four to walk with, the two foremost serving instead of Hands, to take up any thing to eat, to clean her Mouth, Eyes, Wings and Body, and for many other Purposes

L L, The two Wings, fastned with strong Joints to the upper Part of the *Thorax*. Many Particulars of their Contexture have been already given, *Fig* 4 *Plate* XX and something further will be said concerning them in the next Figure of the present Plate

The hinder or Tail-Part of a most lovely shining Blue, looking exactly like polished Steel, brought to that curious Colour by annealing, and seems like a kind of Armour, thickly beset with such-like Bristles as grow upon its Back

In this and most Kinds of Flies, the Female is furnished with a moveable Tube at the End of her Tail, by extending of which she can convey her Eggs into convenient Holes and Receptacles, either in Flesh or such other Matters as may afford the young ones proper Nourishment From the Eggs come forth minute *Worms* or *Maggots*, which after feeding a while in a voracious manner, arriving at their full Growth, become transformed into brown *Aurelias*, whence after some time longer they issue perfect Flies.

Upon opening a Fly, numberless Veins may be discovered dispersed over the Surface of its Intestines, for the Veins being blackish, and the Intestines white, they are plainly visible by the Microscope, though two hundred thousand times slenderer than the Hairs of a Man's Beard According to Mr LEEUWENHOEK †, the Diameter of four hundred and fifty such minute Veins were about equal to the Diameter of a single Hair of his Beard : And consequently two hundred thousand of them put together would be about the Bigness of such a Hair

This Creature is extremely nimble and quick-sighted, so that it will commonly escape, though you approach it ever so cautiously and swiftly. On seeing any thing it fears, it squats down, to be the readier for its Rise, and is very vigorous in its Motions, as well as impudent, for it will return several times to the same Place after being driven away.

Was it not from a preposterous Humour in Mankind, that constantly inclines us to despise and overlook whatever is continually before us, we should often divert ourselves with observing the pretty Actions of this little familiar Animal, which are very well worth our Notice. To see it, like a little Bird, taking its Flight about us, and when it thinks fit to settle, using its Fore-feet to clean its Body, Head and Wings, and afterwards rubbing them backwards and forwards one against the other, to clear away any Dirt they may have contracted in making the other Parts clean : To see its Manner of feeding, the Motions of all its little Members, and the delicate Structure and Contrivance of them : To see all this, I say, and consider how many Veins, Arteries, Nerves, and Muscles, must be employed to give Motion to, and furnish all these Parts with animal Spirits and circulating Fluids, and reflect on the Contexture and Delicacy of Vessels so inconceivably minute, must fill the Mind with Delight and Admiration.

As corrupting Animal Bodies afford the most kindly Nourishment to its Young, it is endued with a wonderful Capacity, either by its Smell, or some other Way, of finding out such Bodies, and laying its Eggs among them.

All the Winter it lies torpid in some Hole or Corner, whence it creeps out at the Return of Spring : But no Cold, nor even being frozen, kills it, for when thawed gently by a Fire, or in the Sun-shine, it revives again : If put into Spirit of Wine, it seems quickly dead, but on taking it out, letting it lie three or four Hours, and then bringing it to a gentle Fire, or putting it in the Heat of the Sun, it will again appear alive

* *Microscope made easy*, p 220   † *Arc Nat* Tom II p 77.

PLATE

A Fly's Wing.

PLATE XXII.   FIG. 2.

A Fly's Wing.

A Fly's Wing,

WE are shewn here the whole of a Fly's Wing, of which we examined the particular Composition in the *Fourth Figure* of the *Twentieth Plate*, whereto we therefore so far refer the Reader , only observing farther on its general Appearance before the Microscope, that it somewhat resembles a *Sea-Fan*, with black Ribs or Fibres dispersed and branched through it ; between which a fine Membrane or Film like a thin Piece of *Muscovy Talc* extends.

It grows from the *Thorax*, a little more towards the 'Head than the Center of the Body's Gravity : But this Excentricity is wonderfully balanced by its expanded Area, and the Center of its Vibration lying much more towards the Tail than the Root of the Wing is.

Our Author tells us, (having made many Trials to find out after what manner the vibrative Motions of a Fly's Wings are performed) that the extreme Limits of the Vibrations were usually about the Length of the Body distant from one another, tho' often shorter, and sometimes longer : That commonly the foremost Limit was a little above the Back, and the hinder somewhat below the Belly , between which two Limits, if one may guess by the Sound, the Wing seemed to move backwards and forwards with an equal Velocity . And these Vibrations between the two Limits are so swift, that 'tis very likely it makes many hundreds, if not thousands, of Vibrations in a Second of Time , so that probably the Wing of a Fly is one of the quickest Vibrations in the World.

Who that considers this can forbear admiring the extreme Vivacity of the *governing Faculty* or *Anima* of the Insect, which is able so to actuate and regulate the Animal Spirits, as to cause each peculiar Organ to move or act not only with so much Quickness, but at the same time with such exact Regularity.

M is a little Body, like in Appearance to a long hanging Drop of some transparent viscid Fluid. This is one of the Ballances or Poises which most Kinds of Flies that have only two Wings are furnished with. It grows out just under the hinder Part of the Root of the Wing, and may be observed constantly to move before it. The Use of these Poises is undoubtedly to keep the Body steady and upright in flying , for if one of them be cut off, the Insect will fly as if one Side was over-balanced, and ere long tumble to the Ground , and if both be taken away, its Flight is aukward and unsteady, manifesting the Want of some necessary and essential Part.

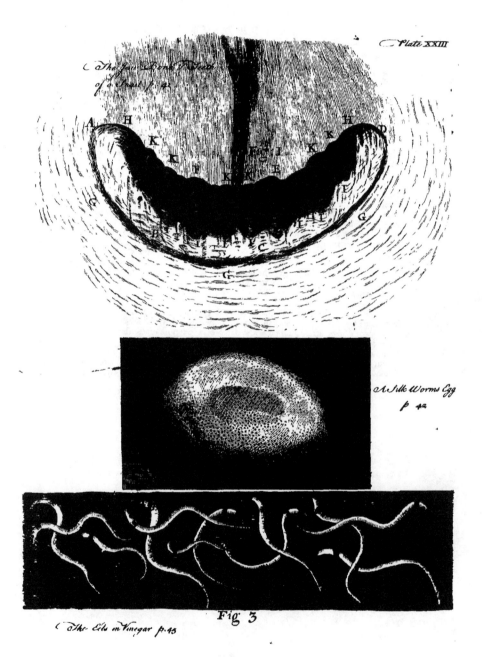

Plate XXIII

The fore Part of a Bee p. 42

A Silk Worms Egg
p 42

The Eels in Vinegar p. 45

Fig 3

An EXPLANATION of the TWENTY-THIRD PLATE.

FIG. 1.

The Teeth of a Snail.

THE upper Jaw-Bone and Teeth of a Garden-Snail are here magnified for our Observation.

The whole was a small bended hard Bone, the Teeth all joining together like the Teeth of a *Rhinoceros*; which perhaps is the only known Animal besides that has them in that manner.

The Part A B C D, which grew out of the upper Chap of the Snail G G G, was found to be much whiter and less furrowed, than the lower and blacker Part of it H I I H K K H, which was shaped exactly like Teeth, the Bone growing thinner and tapering towards an Edge at K K K. It seemed to have nine Teeth or prominent Parts, some smaller than others, but all joined together by thinner interposing Parts of the same Bone

This very Snail, just before its Dissection, was seen feeding on a Rose-Leaf, and biting out half round Pieces, not unlike the Figure of a Capital C, nor much differing from it in Bigness.

Though a Snail is known to every Body, there are some Particulars belonging to it may not be amiss to mention. Its Way of moving from place to place, though destitute of Feet, is effected by two large muscular Skins, that are lengthned by letting out, after which, their Fore-part is shortned into Folds, and the hinder Part falls into the same Contraction. Then the Fore-part extends, and draws along the Shell   A glutinous Slime emitted from the Body, enables it, at the same time, to adhere firmly and securely to all Kinds of Surfaces, which is an Advantage few Animals that have Feet can pretend to.

Snails are oviparous, but their Way of Coupling is extraordinary. They are all Hermaphrodites, each possessing the generative Parts of both Sexes, which are employed mutually *in Coitu*   These Parts are situated on the Left-side of the Head, and are only discoverable when they are generating, which usually engages them about twelve Hours, and from which they can hardly be separated without hurting the Parts.

The Manner of their coming together, as related by Dr. LISTER, is very extraordinary -- -When they are disposed to approach each other, they signify their mutual Inclinations in a Manner peculiar to themselves. One launches against the other a kind of little Dart, which has four Wings or minute Edges. The Weapon flies from the Animal who shot it, and either lodges in the other, or falls down by him, after making a slight Wound, upon which, this Creature in his turn dispatches another Dart at the Aggressor   But this little Combat is immediately succeeded by a Reconciliation. The Substance of the Dart is like Horn, and the Animals are stocked with them at the Seasons when these Approaches are made, and which happen each Year thrice in six Weeks, or once every fifteen Days Some Days after, each makes its Way into the Earth, and lays its Eggs in Knots of about thirty in Number, near four Inches deep. The Place they chuse is commonly moist and shady. In about a Month the Eggs are hatched, and the young Snails appear above Ground, with their Shells compleatly formed, of a Minuteness proportionable to their little Bodies and the Dimensions of the Eggs that inclosed them.   * These Shells increase from time to time by the Addition of new Circles, but continue always to be the Center even when the Animals are arrived at their full Growth. If they are broken by any Accident, a slimy Exsudation from the Body repairs them again in a few Days.

'Tis said no Cold either of Nature or Art can freeze the Juice of Snails, which perhaps is owing to its Viscosity, as we find the Berries of *Misletoe*, whose Juices are of that Quality, are so far from being frozen by, that they ripen in the coldest Weather.

A Snail's Heart may be found just against a round Hole near its Neck, which opens and shuts as it either stands still or moves, and is supposed by Dr. HARVEY to be the Place of its Respiration. It will sometimes beat a Quarter of an Hour after Dissection But without that Trouble it may be seen by the Microscope through the transparent Shell of a new-hatched Snail performing its Contractions and Dilatations with the utmost Regularity

* *Malpigh. Anat. de Colih.   Memoires de l'Academie des Sciences*, 1709

M   The

The Guts are of a pure green Colour after feeding, and appear branched over with little capillary white Veins It has also Liver, Spleen, Stomach, Mouth, and Teeth (which have been just now described) and semi-spherical Eyes at the Tips of the Horns, which if cut off and examined look like large blue Beads.

PLATE XXIII. FIG. 2.

The Egg of a Silk-Worm.

Silk-Worm's Egg

THE minute Egg of this little Animal, when magnified by Glasses, exhibits an Appearance well worthy our Admiration, for innumerable Cavities or Hollows, extremely small, with Risings interposed, somewhat resembling those on a Poppy-Seed, overspread its whole Surface But the Cavities and Ridges here are less an hundred times than those on the Seeds of Poppy, and not distinguishable without a good Instrument and a good Light.

Shell

When the Young is hatched, and the Shell broke, it seems no thicker, in proportion to its Bigness, than the Egg-shell of a Goose or Hen It looks then of a pure white, and so transparent, that none of the little Pits on its Surface can be discerned, without great Difficulty . But a most delicate thin Film may be discovered lining its Inside, in the manner of large Eggs , the Shell itself is very brittle

The Figure of these Eggs is not exactly round, but somewhat flatted both on the upper and under Side , and the included Insect may be discovered lying coiled near the Edges of it But several other Sorts of Moths lay Eggs exactly globular, with Surfaces perfectly smooth and polished , and there is no less Variety in the Eggs of Insects than in those of Birds

These Eggs hatch sooner or later in the Spring, according to the Warmth of the Weather , and may be forwarded very much by keeping them in a certain Degree of Heat. The young Brood appears at first to be a Number of black hairy little Catterpillars, bearing not the least Resemblance to the Forms they afterwards assume. As therefore the Manner of their Changing is wonderful, and many may be desirous to see it with their own Eyes, some short Directions how to feed and manage them, though not altogether requisite in this Place, will not, 'tis hoped, be judged impertinent

Directions how to breed Silk-worms in *England*.

IN *China*, *India*, and some other hot Countries, the Silk-worms live abroad in the open Air, upon Mulberry-Trees propagated in great Abundance for their Reception On these they feed, expatiating in full Liberty, till they inclose themselves in Balls of Silk, curiously fastned to the Branches, and appearing like golden Apples amidst the beautiful Green that embellishes and contrasts them. Here too they affix their Eggs on Parts of the Tree proper for their Preservation, with a Sort of Glew bestowed on them by Providence for that purpose , where they remain secure all the Autumn and Winter-Season, nor begin to hatch till the young expanding Leaves afford them abundant Sustenance

But in our cold Climate, these Creatures must be treated in a quite different manner, and preserved in Houses with a great deal more Care and Trouble As soon as they are hatched, which is commonly some time in *May*, and before the *Mulberry* Leaves come out, the Papers on which the Eggs are laid with us, are to be placed in a Sheet of stiff Writing-Paper, (turned up on every side in the Fashion of a Dripping-Pan) laying lightly upon them the young tender Leaves of *Lettice*. On these they will crawl and feed , and a fresh Supply must be given them as often as the Leaves grow withered , taking care to help some of them off the withered Leaves by the Assistance of a Pin, without which many will be thrown away or destroyed For a Thread which issues from their Mouths, and by sticking to whatever it touches, preserves them from the Danger of falling, sometimes binds them down so fast to the old Leaves, that they become unable to quit them without a little Assistance

In a few Days, the little Catterpillar that was black at first, approaches nearer to an Ashen Grey Its Coat appears ragged, the Animal casts it off, and is seen in a new Habit. It increases in Bigness, and grows whiter, with a little Tendency to green Some Days after this, it forbears eating, and sleeps almost two Days, at the End whereof it seems agitated and convulsed, and grows almost red with the Violence of its Struggles The
Skin

Skin wrinkles, shrinks into Folds, and by little and little the Insect gets it off him with his Feet.

It appears now in its third Habit, and so different are its Head, its Colour, and its whole Form, that one would take it for another Creature. It feeds again some Days, and is then seized with a new Lethargy and Convulsions, and flings off another Skin, after which its Appetite returns, and it feeds voraciously, growing continually larger and whiter, with a delicate Smoothness and Transparency of its Skin, which foretells the Time of its Spinning being near at hand. It then leaves off feeding for the Remainder of its Life, and seeks some Corner where it begins to form its Web.

But to return to our feeding them with *Lettice*-Leaves, which must be their Provision till the *Mulberry* Trees shoot out. Care must be taken that the Leaves be perfectly dry when put to them, (for any Moisture does them Harm,) and that they be not given in too great Quantity at once, but fresh and often.

As the Creatures grow they must be divided into two or more Dripping-pan-formed Papers, in proportion to their Number; observing, during the whole Course of their Changes, never to crowd Multitudes of them together, for doing so breeds an Infection sometimes amongst them, that carries off a great many.

When they begin to feed on Mulberry-Leaves, (which should be given them as soon as such Leaves can be got) they will thrive much faster than before. But then they must never be left without Food, for as they live but a short Period before they begin to spin, and after that live almost as long without eating any thing, they make the best Use of their Time, and are feeding continually till their Changes come. A great deal of their Welfare depends likewise on keeping them perfectly clean and sweet, by clearing the Papers of their Dung and the Remains of their Leaves, as often as there is Occasion.

When they arrive at their full Growth, and forsaking their Food begin to spin in some Corner of the Dripping-Pan, each of them must be put in a little Paper-Cone of about an Inch and half Diameter at its open End. These Cones should be sewed together in Couples, and hung across a Pack-thread Line, or fastned to it singly, as your Number or Fancy shall direct.

The Silk-Worm's Manner of making Silk.

LET us now behold this industrious Animal at work, a Sight which must fill the attentive Observer with an equal Mixture of Delight and Wonder. After surveying the Dimensions of her Paper-Cone, she begins to form her Web, applying her Mouth to different Parts of the Paper, and then pulling her Head away with a slow but equal Motion. To explain the Meaning of this, it is necessary to take notice, that immediately below her Mouth are a Couple of little Holes, which are the Outlets of a long and slender Bag filled with a kind of yellow viscid Juice or Gum. Wherever the little Creature applies these two Openings, the viscid Juice adheres, and when the Head is drawn back, continuing to flow through them, receives their Form (as Wire does from the Hole it is pulled through) and lengthens into a double Thread, which instantly losing the Fluidity of the Juice composing it, obtains the Consistence of Silk. These two Threads she unites in one, glewing them together with a Sort of Fingers on her Fore-Paws; and at the Beginning of her Work fastens them here and there as it were at random, and soon encompasses herself with a loose and hasty Covering, just sufficient (was she abroad) to defend her from the Rain. Within this she weaves another Case, made of the finest Silk, disposed with the utmost Regularity, and rendered so perfectly compact as to prevent any Admission of the Air. Nor is she contented with these two Coverings, but forms within them both a kind of Shell, composed of Silk and Glew, and resembling a very strong Stuff, which not only can repel Water and Air, but be a good Security against the Rigour of the severest Frosts.

Thus defended from Danger, she undergoes a most amazing *Metamorphosis*, relinquishes intirely her former Figure, and appears, if taken out of these Cases, a crustaceous Acornlike Body, having neither Head, Legs, Eyes, or any distinct Part, and but very few Signs of Life. In short, she becomes a *Nymph* or *Chrysalis*.

She continues thus, seemingly dead and intombed, for a Fortnight, three Weeks, or sometimes a longer Time, when she obtains a glorious Resurrection, and comes out provided with four beauteous Wings, of a Cream Colour, almost white, with regular and uniform Lines of a very light grey on each, and covered all over with delicate downy Plumes. She has two fine Eyes, a Pair of Horns exquisitely branched, and her Body and six Legs are every where adorned with Hairs and Feathers of a most curious Structure,

i   and

and as different from one another as the Feathers on the different Parts of the Bodies of Birds are. In ſhort, ſhe becomes a very pretty Butterfly or Moth.

But it may be enquired how this tender Animal is able to force a Paſſage through its three Coverings, *viz.* the Shell, the Silk, and the looſer Web juſt now deſcribed, and indeed its Proviſion and Forecaſt for this Purpoſe deſerve our Attention and Admiration. Theſe Coverings are faſhioned like a Pigeon's Egg, ſharper at one End than the other; and towards this Extremity, the Worm, as if conſcious here muſt be its Paſſage out, neither interweaves its Silk, nor applies its Glew, as in every Part beſides. Oppoſite to this Point the Head is conſtantly placed in its *Nympha* State, and as ſoon as its Formation into a Butterfly is compleated, its Horns, Head and Feet extend themſelves againſt this Part, which not being cemented, gradually gives Way, and affords an Opening for its coming out.

This is their natural Courſe, but as they conſtantly diſcharge from their Bodies, a large Quantity of a reddiſh-brown Liquor, when they firſt appear in the Fly-State, which ſtains and damages the Silk; thoſe that keep them either for Profit or Amuſement, uſually prevent this, either by winding off their Silk before they are ready for this Change, or if that cannot be done, by expoſing them to the intenſe Heat of the Sun, or a Fire, for ſome Hours, to kill them in their Caſes : reſerving only ſome few for Breed.

How to wind off Silk.

T HE Pods may eaſily be wound off, if after pulling away the looſe outward Covering, (which may be ſpun like Flax for ordinary Purpoſes) they be put into warm Water, for that diſſolves the Gum, and ſets the Silk at liberty to be unravelled from End to End; and ſome Spirit of Wine added to the Water makes the Gum diſſolve ſtill more readily   Ten or a Dozen Threads of as many Pods may be wound off together very conveniently either in Skeens or Balls, till we come to the innermoſt Covering or Shell, which is of a whiter Colour, much more gummy, and a Sort of Silk but of little Uſe or Virtue. It is therefore commonly the Way to cut them open, and take out the included *Nymphæ*, which being then naked ſhould be laid on dry freſh Bran till they become Butterflies.

Some Ladies pull away the looſe Silk, cut out the *Nymphæ*, and dye the Pods of all Colours in great Variety of Shades, after which they compoſe with them moſt beautiful Noſegays of artificial Flowers.

The Largeneſs of its Size diſtinguiſhes the Female even in its *Nympha* State, but that Diſtinction is ſtill more evident after they appear as Flies. The Males are exceeding lively and ſalacious, endeavouring continually, by their noiſy Flutterings and wanton Motions, to raiſe Deſire in the Females. The Coitus continues ſometimes ſeveral Hours, during which the Body of the Female may be obſerved to ſwell and enlarge. ſoon after ſhe begins to depoſite her Eggs, and perhaps goes on to do ſo from time to time till ſhe has laid above five hundred

As ſoon as they become Butterflies, 'tis beſt to put them in ſuch Paper Dipping-Pans as when they were Catterpillars, for they will rarely get over the Sides of the Paper, and it is very convenient for them to ſtick their Eggs to. The Females are full of Eggs even in the *Nympha* State, and will lay, though no Male comes near them, but ſuch Eggs are unprolific. When firſt the Eggs are laid, their Colour is a Pale-Lemon, but they ſoon grow darker, and after a Week or two appear of a Lead-Colour   Thoſe that continue yellow will never produce any thing.

Their Semen full of Animalcules.

U PON gently ſqueezing the Tail of a *Male-Fly* for a little while, a ſmall Drop of a whitiſh brown Liquor will be ſquirted from it, which diluted with a little warm Water, and examined by the Microſcope, appears crowded with Animalcules, four times as long as broad, with Backs thicker than their Bellies, like the Shape of a Trout *   But this muſt be done before the Male has been coupled with the Female, for nothing is to be got from it afterwards.

After the Females have done laying they grow languid and die in a Day or two, and the Males do not long ſurvive them. The Papers whereon the Eggs are laid may be folded up and kept in any ſafe Place till the following Spring, when they will certainly be hatched, ſooner or later, according to the Warmth of the Seaſon.

The

* *Vid. Leeuwenb. Arc. Nat. Tom.* I *P.* II *p* 42*1*

The exquifite Finenefs of the Silk fpun by this little Creature, well deferves our Notice. A Pod being wound off, was found to contain nine hundred and thirty Yards : But it is proper to obferve, that as two Threads are glewed together by the Worm through the whole Length of the Silk, it really makes double the above Number, or one thoufand eight hundred and fixty Yards, which being weighed with the utmoft Exactnefs, were found no heavier than two Grains and a half.

The whole *Butterfly* and *Moth* Tribe undergo the fame Changes as the *Silk-worm* does, though with fome Variation, as to Time, and Place, and Manner. Some fpin filky Cafes like them , others wrap themfelves up in Leaves, which they cement together by a gummy Exfudation from their own Bodies , fome defcend into the Ground, form Cafes of Earth, and wait their Changes there , and others again only hang themfelves by the Tail in fome fhelter'd Corner, where from Catterpillars they become *Aurelias*, and from *Aurelias*, *But-terflies* There is likewife a confiderable Difference as to Time, fome paffing through all their Changes in a few Weeks, and fome taking up above a Year. But they all agree in proceeding from the Egg a *Caterpillar*, and becoming afterwards a *Nymph*, *Chryfalis*, or *Aurelia*, and at laft a *Moth* or *Butterfly*.

Some few Lines from a Poem before quoted, called the UNIVERSE, expreffive of this wonderful Change, will not, 'tis hoped, be thought improper here.

See, to the Sun the Butterfly *difplays*
Its glitt'ring Wings, and wantons in his Rays ·
In Life exulting, o'er the Meadows flies,
Sips from each Flower, and breathes the vernal Skies.
Where Love directs, a Libertine, it roves,
And courts the Fair Ones through the verdant Groves ;
While its rich Plumes, in graceful Order, fhow
The various Glories of the painted Bow.

How beauteous now ! how chang'd fince Yefterday !
When on the Ground, a crawling Worm it lay,
Where every Foot might tread its Soul away.
Who rais'd it thence, and bid it range the Skies ?
Gave its rich Plumage, and its brilliant Dyes ?

'Twas GOD :----Its GOD and thine, O Man ! and He
In this thy Fellow-Creature lets Thee fee,
That wond'rous Change which is ordain'd for Thee !

Thou too fhalt leave thy reptile Form behind,
And mount the Skies, a pure ætherial Mind,
There range among the Stars, all bright and unconfin'd.

PLATE XXIII. FIG. 3.

Eels in Vinegar.

THESE little Animals wherewith Vinegar is fometimes abundantly ftored, very much refemble an Eel in Shape, and in the Nimblenefs of their Motion , with this Difference, however, that the wriggling Motion of their Bodies feems to be upwards and downwards only ; whereas that of Eels is only fideways: Their Nofe is likewife fomething fharper than the Eel's, and more opake than the reft of the Body, as is fhewn at A.

Dr. HOOKE obferved alfo a dark Part at B, which he imagined to be the Gills, as it appeared at a fmall Diftance from the Nofe . And from this Part the Body grows conti-nually tapering to the Tip of the Tail C.

The progressive Motion of these Creatures in the Vinegar is exceeding slow, notwithstanding the continual waving and wriggling of their Bodies, which may reasonably be imputed to the Resistance of the Fluid, as the Superficies of their minute Bodies is so very great in proportion to their Bulk

These Animals immediately die if the Vinegar be a little heated, but they do not suffer much by Cold, for Dr. Power * says, he froze artificially a Glass Jarr-full of Vinegar replete with them, into a Mass of Ice, yet when it was thawed, they all appeared as brisk as ever · Nay, he adds, that having exposed them a whole Night to a keen Frost, upon thawing the Ice next Morning, they seemed to have received no manifest Injury, notwithstanding that long and strong Conglaciation ---He tells us likewise, that he filled an Essence-Glass half with the said Vinegar, and half with Oil which floated on it ; and observed in frosty Weather, when the Vinegar was congealed, that all the little Eels ran up into the super-incumbent Oil, and would not return till some Warmth was applied to the Vinegar, but if that was a little warmed, they immediately descended into it again

Some Experiments on freezing Vinegar, with these Eels in it, were made about a Year ago, and communicated to the *Royal Society* by Dr HENRY MILES, F R S. the Result whereof was, upon several Trials, that the greatest Number were found irrecoverably dead, tho' many endured the being frozen, recovered after a little while, and appeared as brisk as ever

Dr HOOKE says, that a Quantity of Vinegar, replete with these Eels, being included in a small Phial, and stopped very close from the ambient Air, all the included Worms in a short time died, as if they had been stifled : But this is not constantly the Case, for the ingenious Observer just now mentioned, had a Couple of Tubes, (of the Sort employed to behold the Circulation of the Blood) both which were full of Vinegar, well stocked with these Eels, and as well stopped with Cork as they could be, the Liquor too reaching so near the Top as just to touch the Cork, and though these were not opened once in a Month, yet they lived, increased greatly, and were surprisingly brisk The Tubes always stood in a Cup-board just over the Fire-Place, and so near it, that they were sensibly warm, there being a constant Fire

The Eels in Paste seem nearly of the same Kind as those in Vinegar The Manner of producing which, and the Way of examining them, may be found in the 81st Page of the *Microscope made easy*

* *Power's Observ* p 35

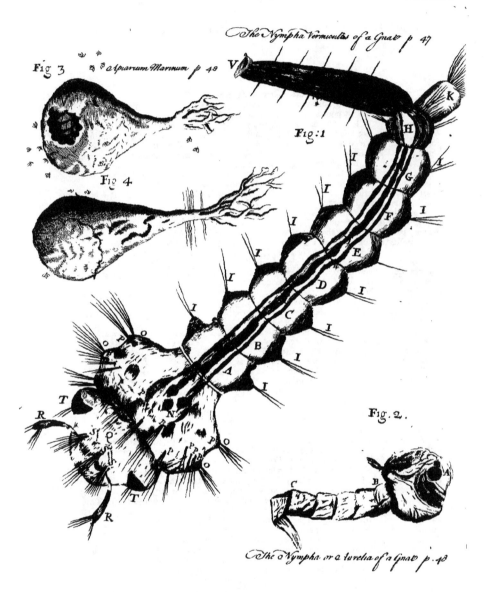

Plate XXIV

Fig 3

Apiarium Marinum p. 48

The Nympha Vermiculus of a Gnat p. 47

Fig: 1

Fig 4

Fig. 2.

The Nympha or Aurelia of a Gnat p. 48

An EXPLANATION of the TWENTY-FOURTH PLATE.

FIG. 1.

The Nymph-Worm of a Gnat.

IT may be requisite towards the better understanding of this Figure, to premise a short Account of the Generation of a Gnat, and the Changes it undergoes Nymph Worm of a Gnat

The Female depofites its Eggs upon the Surface of the Waters, by dipping down its Tail, and emitting a Quantity (large in Proportion to the Fly) of a Spawn or Jelly-like Subftance, which it conftantly faftens to fome Weed, or fuch like kind of Thing In this Jelly, which is tranfparent, and at firft floats upon the Water, the minute Eggs are ranged, fometimes in fingle, and fometimes in double Rows, not ftrait, but waving, though very regular and exact.

These Eggs become hatched after fome Time, and produce fmall reddifh Maggots, which finking to the Bottom of the Water with fome of the Slime wherein they were envelop'd, faften to Stones or other Bodies, and make themfelves little Cafes, which they can creep out of or retire into as they find Occafion

When they have continued thus as long as Providence has appointed, they become changed into the Figure under Examination (which we term the *Nympha Vermiculus*) are very active, and fwim about the Water with brifk jerking Motions

From this they change into the State reprefented by the next Figure in this Plate, which may be called the *Aurelia* or *Nymph*, and out of that they proceed *Gnats*

Authors are a little obfcure in their Accounts of the Changes this Creature undergoes, and not quite confiftent with one another. SWAMMERDAM gives two Figures anfwerable to the two we find in this Plate, calling the firft the *Worm*, and the other the *Nympha* of the Gnat, but mentions not the real *Worm*, which 'tis therefore probable he had not obferved. On the other Hand, our ingenious Countryman DERHAM is very full as to the *Worm*, but evidently confounds together into one the *two States* defcribed and pictured by both SWAMMERDAM and Dr HOOKE, and fpeaks only of three States ; whereas the Progreffion of the Gnat from the Egg is, firft, into a *Worm*, which may be called its *Vermicular-State*, then into the Figure before us, or its *Nympha Vermicular-State*, thirdly, into the fecond Figure of this Plate, not improperly its *Aurelia* or *Nympha-State*, and laftly, into the *Gnat*, or its *Mature State*

The Way being thus cleared before us, we come to defcribe this *Nympha-Vermiculus*, a Creature frequently met with in Ponds, Ditches, Cifterns, and all Repofitories of Water during moft of the Summer Seafon Its general Form will beft be underftood by the Picture we are going to examine, wherein A B C D E F G H reprefent the Belly Part, confifting of eight diftinct Divifions, from the midft of each whereof iffue out on either Side two or three little Hairs or Briftles, I I I I, &c.

The Tail is compofed of two Parts, of a very different Figure and Ufe The Part K, whofe End is covered with Hairs, ferves both as Oars and Rudder, enabling this little Creature, together with the frifking and bending of its Body nimbly too and fro, not only to move about with great Agility, but to fteer itfelf whither it pleafes

L fhews the other Part of the Tail, which feems to be a Continuation of, and may be term'd a ninth Divifion of its Belly Many fingle Briftles grow from it on every Side, and quite to the Extremity thereof V, from that orbicular Part of the Body N, which appears to be the Stomach, a Gut extends along through the whole Belly This Gut is of a darkifh Colour, and difpofed in the Manner diftinguifhed by the Letters M M M, &c A periftaltic Motion therein agitated a Kind of black Subftance, very remarkably, upwards and downwards from the Stomach to the Anus Lice, Gnats, and feveral other tranfparent Infects may be obferved to have the like periftaltic Motion

O O O O the Cheft or Thorax, fhort, thick, fhelly, and pretty tranfparent, with in which the Beating of the Heart (which is white, as is alfo the Blood of this and moft other Infects) and feveral other Motions may be difcerned by the Microfcope

The Cheft is ornamented and defended, in feveral Places, with Tufts of ftrong Briftles, *p p p p p* Q fhews the Head, broad, fhort, and cruftaceous, having three Tufts of the fame kind of Briftles on its Forehead or upper Part, S S S

T T are two fine large black Eyes, whofe Surfaces are fmooth, and without the leaft Appearance of being pearled or granulated, as we fhall find them in the next Figure and Change of this Animal I

R R

R R a Pair of Horns refembling thofe of an Ox inverted, with Briftles at their Tops, and feeming to be hollow   Thefe are moveable every Way, and may probably be of confiderable Service to the Infect

Its Mouth is pretty large, in the Fafhion of a Crab's or Lobfter's, and it may frequently be feen feeding on fome minute Subftances in the Water

This Creature moves in the Water with its Tail forwards, jerking itfelf along by the Frifking to and fro of the Tuft growing out from the Stump thereof   It has alfo another Motion, more refembling that of other Animals, and with its Head foremoft, for by the opening and fhutting of its Jaws, it finks gently towards the Bottom of the Water, and prefently afterwards feems as it were to eat its Way up again

When the Body ceafes to move, the Tail being higher than the Water wherein it fwims, or than any other Part of the Infect, prefently buoys it up to the Surface of the Water, where it hangs fufpended with its Head always downwards; for the Brufh it the Tail being fmeared over with an oily Fluid, ferves like a Cork to keep it above Water, and it that Oil begins to dry, the Creature by drawing the Tail through its Mouth fheds thereon a new Supply, and enables it to hang to the Top of the Water, or fteer where it pleafes, without being wetted or damaged by it.

PLATE XXIV. FIG. 2.

The Nympha or Aurelia of the Gnat.

Nymph of the Gnat

THE Animal juft now defcribed, after about three Weeks, affumes a Form very different from what it had before, and agreeable to what we fee before us   The Head and Body become larger and deeper, but not broader, the Belly and hinder Parts appear more flender, and feem coiled about the Body in the Fafhion reprefented by the pricked Lines in the Picture

In this new State, the Head and Horns, which before hung downwards in the Water, rife uppermoft to the Surface, and what is very remarkable, the Infect becomes now fufpended from the Top of the Water by its Horns *, as it was lately by its Tail. The whole Bulk of the Body is alfo evidently higher, for when by being frighted it frifks out its Tail, as B C reprefents, and thereby finks below the Surface and towards the Bottom, it re-afcends much more fwiftly than in its former State

If its Progrefs be now obferved from Time to Time, its Body will be found gradually to inlarge, Nature fitting it by Degrees for that Element of which it muft quickly be an Inhabitant   The Microfcope alfo fhews, that its Eyes are now pearled like the Eyes of Gnats (vid A) not fmooth as they were before   And that this Club Head really contains the Thorax and Wings of the future Gnat   A little longer Obfervation will fhew it fwimming partly above and partly below the Surface of the Water, and though it may then be made to plunge down by touching it with any Thing, it inftantly comes up again, and appears in its former Pofture

And now, if we have Patience to watch it narrowly, we fhall be rewarded with the fatisfaction of beholding the Head and Body of a Gnat beginning to fhew themfelves above the Surface of the Water   We fhall fee its Legs gradually drawn out, firft the two foremoft, then the others, and foon after, its whole Body will appear rifing out of the Hufk or Cafe perfect and intire   We fhall fee it difengage itfelf from this Cafe, and ftand on its Legs upon the Top of the Water, there by Degrees try the Activity of its Wings, and in a few Minutes fly away a compleat Gnat.

PLATE XXIV. FIG. 3 and 4

Apiarium Marinum.

THESE two Figure are given from Piso Natural Hiftory of Brafil, in the fecond Chapter of his fourth Book, where fpeaking of Sea Productions that bear fome near Refemblance to Productions upon Land, he tells the Story of a Fifherman, whofe Hook being entangled contrary to his Expectation, on a rocky Shallow not far from Parnambuque brought up with it, on his pulling it out of the Water, Sponges, Coral, and Sea-weed, inftead of Fifh

He

Plate XXV

The Tufted or Brush-horn'd Gnat p.49.

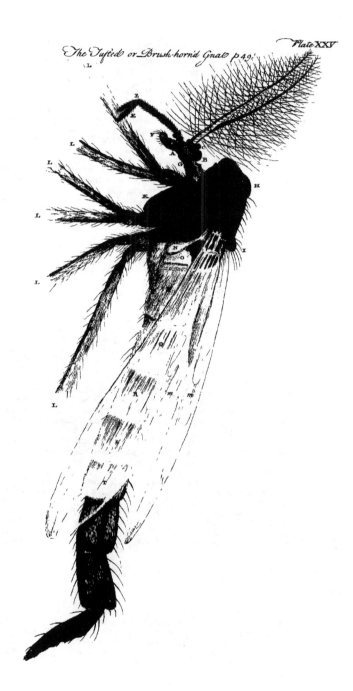

He took Notice, amongst the rest, of a little odd-shaped Plant, about half a Foot in Length, with a soft, spungy, roundish Body, enlarging from the Bottom upwards after the Fashion of a Pear ; and having short Roots, which had fastened it to the Rock. The Inside of it was composed of wonderful little Cells and Hollows, and its Surface was all over covered with a tenacious sticky Matter, resembling the Glew of Bees On the Top was a wide and deep Opening or Entrance (as is shewn in the third Figure) so that it might properly be called *Apiarium Marinum*, or a *Sea-Bee's Nest* , for as soon as it was brought to Land, it swarmed with little b'ewish Worms, which by the Heat of the Sun were changed afterwards into small black Flies, or rather Bees , but they flying all away, nothing can be asserted as to their making Honey However, as the little Cells or Combs and waxy Matter of Bees were evidently there, without doubt the Substance of the Honey itself, or whatever else is contained within them, will be discovered by the Divers, when they shall observe these Bees-Nests more curiously, and thoroughly examine them at different Seasons of the Year, in the Places where they are produced

This is the Substance of Piso's Account, which the two Figures before us represent , and from thence Dr Hooke takes Occasion to enquire, " Whether the Hulk or Case " was a Plant, growing before of itself at the Bottom of the Sea, out of whose Putri- " faction these strange Kind of Maggots might be generated? or whether the Seed " of certain Bees, sinking to the Bottom, might there naturally form itself that vege- " table Hive, and take root? or whether it might not be placed there by some diving " Fly? or whether it might not be some peculiar Propriety of that Plant whereby it " might ripen, or form its vegetable Juice into an Animal Substance? or whether it " may not be of the Nature of a Spunge, or rather a Spunge in the Nature of this?"

***

An EXPLANATION of the TWENTY-FIFTH PLATE.

The tufted or Brush-horned Gnat.

HAVING treated so fully on the Generation and Changes of a Gnat, in de- Brush-horned scribing the first Figure of the last Plate, there is little to do here but to shew Gnat the several Parts of that Animal in its perfect State, as its Picture now lies before us

Dr. DERHAM says *, he observed near forty distinct Species of Gnats about *Up-minster* in *Essex*, and doubtless there are many Sorts beside, but none amongst them all is perhaps more beautiful or remarkable than the Gnat we are now surveying, which is the Male of one of these Species.

The Head A is extremely small in Proportion to its Body, and composed chiefly of two Clusters of pearled Eyes of a greenish Colour, one of which Clusters is shewn at B, whose Pearls or little Eyes are curiously ranged like those of large Flies.

Just over, and somewhat between these Eyes, on the Forehead of the Animal, are a Couple of small black Balls, whereof one is expressed at C, out of which issue two long Horns D, tapering and jointed like the Horns of a Lobster ' From the several Joints of these Horns Multitudes of small stiff Hairs issue on every Side, in a very regular and beautiful Order, making the Whole appear like the Plant *Equisetum*, or *Horse-Tail*. There are also two other jointed and bristled Horns or Feelers, standing before the others, and projecting forwards, such as E E, under which lies the Proboscis F, being a Case covered with long Scales, and concealed under the Gnat's Throat when not made use of. Its Side opens, and four Darts are thrust out thence, occasionally, one whereof, though exceedingly minute, serves for a Sheath to the other thrice. The Sides of them are extremely sharp, and they are barbed towards the Point, whose Fineness is inexpressible, and scarcely to be discerned by the greatest Magnifier When a Gnat finds any tender Fruits or Liquors that it likes, it sucks them through the outer Case, without employing the Darts at all , but if it meets with Flesh, or any Body whose Contexture denies Admittance to the Case, it stings very severely, then sheaths its Weapons in their Scabbard, and through it sucks up the Juices flowing from the Wound.

This small Head with the Ornamental and other Parts thereto belonging, is fastened by a short Neck G, to the Middle of the Thorax, which is large in Proportion to the

O   Animal,

Animal, and of the Shape reprefented H I K: It is perfectly cruftaceous, and befet with little ftiff Hairs or Briftles, inftead of Feathers, and from the under Part thereof proceed fix hairy Legs L L L L, &c each having fix Joints, and at the End two little Claws. Thefe Legs are very long and flender, and could not therefore be given in the Drawing · Their Feet are all over feathered, in a Manner refembling a Fifh's Scales, with Abundance of little black Hairs interfperfed, and appearing ftubborn like Hog's Briftles

From the upper and pofterior Part of the Thorax grow out a Pair of tranfparent, flender, oblong Wings *m m*, whofe Edges are furrounded with a Fringe of Feathers, and under each Wing appears a Poife or Ballance N, having a round Knob at its Extremity, which leffens by Degrees into a fmall Stem, and again grows bigger near its Infertion under the Wing Thefe little Bodies vibrate to and fro very nimbly when the Creature moves its Wings, and move fometimes even when the Wings are quiet, but commonly foretel the Motion of the Wings to follow. As to their Ufe, fee p 40

The Belly or Tail-part is long in Proportion to the Animal, and compofed of nine *Annuli*, or Partitions, fhelly, and armed with fhort Briftles, as well as adorned with Feathers, moft curioufly difpofed in Rows Six of the Divifions O P Q R S T are tranfparent, and in them the periftaltic Motions of the Inteftines are very diftinguifhable. A fmall, clear, white Part is alfo more particularly remarkable at V, which may be feen beating like the Heart of fome larger Animal.

The other three Divifions W X Y are opake, and in the laft of them are fhewn the Figure and Situation of the *Anus*.

An EXPLANATION of the TWENTY-SIXTH PLATE.

The Great-bellyed or Female Gnat.

Greatbellyed Gnat

THE Shape of this Gnat is very different from the preceding, and its Belly, Cheft, Wings, and every other Part larger, as is commonly the Cafe of the Female in all the Tribes of flying Infects Two Pair of Horns appear on the Head of this as well as of the Male, but both Pair here are nearly of the fame Length, whereas in that the brufhy Horns are much longer than the other two; and thefe Horns which in the Male are brufhy and full of Joints, are in the Female only befet with fhort ftrong Briftles, and have much fewer Articulations.

The Thorax Part of this, as well as of the other, has a very ftrong and fhelly Back-piece, which reaches alfo on either Side its Legs: Several jointed Pieces of Shell-work are likewife curioufly and conveniently difpofed about its Wings, and ferve at the fame Time to give them both Strength and Motion

Dr HOOKE permitted one of thefe Infects to penetrate the Skin of his Hand with its Probofcis, and fuck out thence as much Blood as it could poffibly contain, whereby it became red and tranfparent, and all this was done without his fuffering any Pain, except while the Probofcis was making its Entrance, which the Doctor ufes as an Argument to prove, that thefe Creatures do not wound the Skin and fuck the Blood out of Enmity and Revenge, but through mere Neceffity, and to fatisfy their Hunger

Plate XXVI

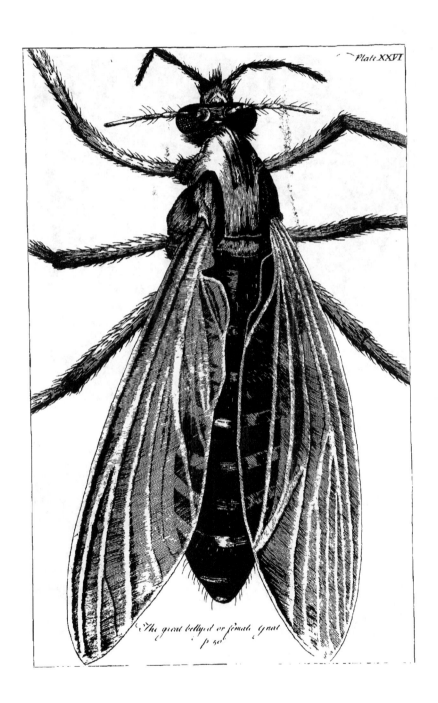

The great bellyed or female Gnat
p 50

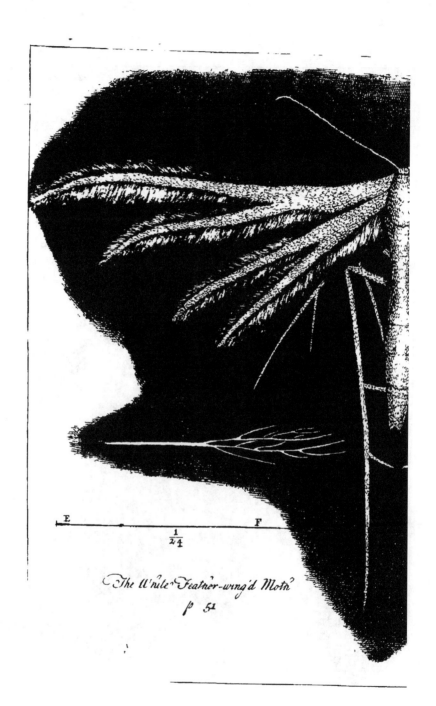

E ———————————————— F

$\frac{1}{2}\frac{1}{4}$

The White Feather-wing'd Moth

p 51

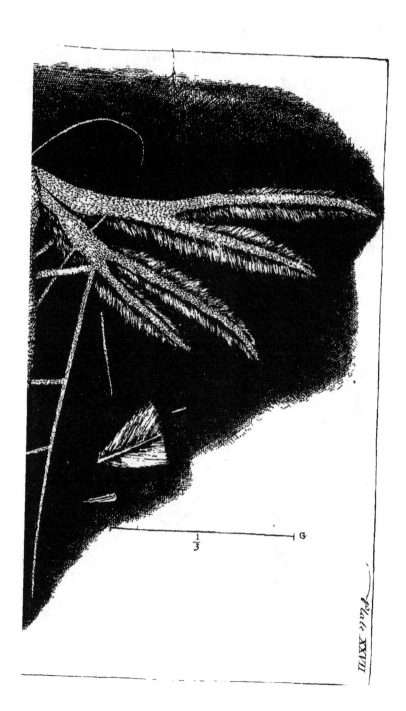

$\frac{1}{3}$

Plate XXVII

An EXPLANATION of the TWENTY-SEVENTH PLATE.

The white Feather-winged Moth.

T H E pretty Object now under Observation was a small white Moth, of a Kind *Feather-* found sometimes upon the Nettle. It had four Wings, each whereof appeared *wing'd* to consist of two long slender Feathers, very elegantly fringed on either Side with ex- *Moth* ceeding fine and small Hairs, proportionable to the Stems out of which they grew, much like the long Wing-feathers of some Birds, their Stems were likewise (as in such Feathers) inclined backwards and downwards, in a Manner which the Drawing shews. Each Wing in the hindermost Pair was about half an Inch in Length, and the fore- most Pair out-measured them by near a Third

This whole Animal, even to the naked Eye, appeared fashioned and contrived with exquisite Regularity and Beauty, but when brought under Examination before the Microscope, every Part of it exhibited an Elegance beyond Description. The Body, Legs, Horns, and Stems of the Wings were covered all over with Feathers of different Shapes and Sizes, appropriated to the particular Places where they grew On the least Touch they came off upon the Fingers, and stuck like a white Powder between the little *Rugae* of the Skin, and being view'd by a Glass that magnified a great deal (of which E F representing the twenty-fourth Part of an Inch, is the Scale; as G, which represents no more than one Third of an Inch, is of a lesser Magnifier) many of them, and especially those interspersed among the Hairs of the Wings, were found to consist of a Stalk or Stem in the Middle, and a brushy Part on each Side, resembling the Figure A

Underneath these Feathers the pretty Insect was covered over with a crusted Shell, extreamly thin and tender.

Surveying its Wings with the greatest Magnifier, the Tufts or Hairs which fringe them as it were along the Edges, appeared to be nothing else but thick-set Rows of little Twigs or Branches, resembling the peeled or whitened Sprigs of Birch wherewith Whisks are made for brushing Beds and Hangings The Form of them is shewn at D

The Stems of the Wings, and the greatest Part of the Body, are covered with Fea- thers, brushy on both Sides like those of a small Bird, as we see at the Letter B. The Horns and small Parts of the Legs were adorned with another Sort, which appeared through the same Microscope of the Shape C.

'Tis uncertain whether the component Parts of these Feathers are the same as those of Birds, but the contrary is most probable, since Providence seems to alter its Method in the Fabrick and Fashion of the Wings of flying Insects, composing some of thin, extended Membranes, as we see in the *Libella* or *Dragon-Fly*, and such Membranes are thick beset with short Hairs or Bristles in others, as the *Flesh-Fly*, &c The Wings of *Moths* and *Butterflies* are covered with small Feathers, both on the upper and under Side, disposed with the utmost Regularity, almost like the Tyles on an House, and adorned with most lovely Colours. The Wings of the present Subject we see divided into four large Feathers: The little *Grey Plume-Moth* has eight or ten such Divisions, each branched somewhat like a Herring-Bone, or a thin-haired Peacock's Feather with the Eye cut off, these shut together, or open Fan-Fashion, all lying under one another when closed, and by each other's Side when expanded. The Beetle Kinds have *Ely-* *trae* or *Case-Wings*, which are hollow Shells in the Form of Butchers Trays, and under them most commonly a Pair of fine filmy membraneous ones are folded up, and secured from being injured by the Earth, wherein these Creatures frequently reside

Now 'tis greatly worth observing, that wherever a Wing consists of discontinued Parts, the Interstices between such Parts are seldom much larger or smaller than what we find between these Brushes, which seems to intimate, that the Particles of Air will not easily, if at all, pass through them, and if so, they serve the Animal as well, nay perhaps better than if they were extended Membranes. Our Author remarks also, that *Bats*, *Dragon-Flies*, *Scarabs*, and such other Creatures as have undivided and smooth Wings, are furnished with stronger Muscles, and move their Wings with much more Strength and Velocity than those *Birds*, *Moths*, and *Butterflies* whose Wings are co- vered with Feathers, and supposes, " The little Ruggedness thereby occasioned may " help their Wings somewhat, by taking better Hold of the Parts of the Air, or not " suffering them so easily to pass by any other Way than one "

I   A N

An EXPLANATION of the TWENTY-EIGHTH PLATE.

FIG. 1.

The Back of the long-legg'd Spider.

Long legg'd Spider.

THE Spider we are about to deſcribe is that found frequently in Fields and Gardens in the Summer and Autumn Seaſons, having eight Legs, extremely long and ſlender, wherewith it ſtrides at a great rate over the Graſs and Herbs. Its Body is very ſmall in proportion to its Legs, in the Center of which it is lifted up on high, as it were on ſo many Stilts. It appears flattiſh, of a grey Colour, and nearly round or oval to the naked Eye, but the Microſcope ſhews the Shell of its Back to be heptangular and ſpeckled. Many know it by the Name of the *Carter, Shepherd-Spider,* or *Field-Spider*

This Spider is moſt remarkable for its Eyes and its long Legs, of both which an Account will be given in due Order The Number of Eyes in Spiders differs according to their different Species, ſome having eight or ten, ſome ſix, and others no more than four placed in their Fore-part or Head, which is without a Neck, but this under Examination has only a ſingle Pair, and thoſe too not ſituated upon the Fore-front, as in other Sorts, but on a Protuberance (which perhaps may be the Head) riſing out of the Middle of the Top of its Back, as in the Figure B B.

PLATE XXVIII. FIG. 2.

The Eyes of the long-legg'd Spider.

Eyes of the long-legg'd Spider.

IN order to give a more ſatisfactory View of theſe Eyes, and their extraordinary Situation, another Drawing is preſented, where the two Eyes B B are placed, back to back, with the tranſparent Parts or Pupils looking on either ſide, but rather forwards than backwards, fixed on the Summit of the Neck C, which is an Eminence on the Middle of the Protuberance D D, and making therewith ſomewhat more than the Height of the tranſverſe Diameter of the Eye

The Structure of theſe Eyes reſembles that of larger *binocular* Animals, having a Cornea very ſmooth and circular, with a black Pupil in the midſt thereof, incircled with a kind of grey *Iris*. The Eyes of other Spiders are immoveable, nor is it poſſible theſe can be turned about in any manner, as the Neck whereon they ſtand is covered and ſtiffened with a cruſty Shell, but this Defect is probably ſupplied by the Roundneſs of the *Cornea*, and the Height of their Situation above the Body, whereby 'tis likely each Eye may perceive, though not diſtinctly, nearly a compleat Hemiſphere, and that having ſo ſmall and round a Body on ſuch long Legs, it is able ſo to wind and turn it as to ſee every thing diſtinct ---All Spiders are without Eyelids, or any Pearling in their Eyes

The beſt Way of coming at a proper Sight of this wonderful Object, is by breaking off all the Legs, as in *Fig.* 1. and then placing it before the Microſcope,

PLATE XXVIII. FIG. 3.

The Belly of the long-legg'd Spider.

Belly of the long legg'd Spider.

WE ſee the ſame Spider turned here with its Belly upwards, to ſhew in what manner the Legs are joined on to the Under-Part of the Thorax And this is all could be given of them in the Figure, their enormous Length rendering it impoſſible to bring them into any ſizeable Drawing, as they appeared magnified by the Microſcope, each Leg of the preſent Spider being above ſixteen times the Length of its whole Body, and there are ſome that have them much longer in proportion. Its Legs are jointed like thoſe of a Crab, but all the Parts of them are prodigiouſly more lengthned out The End of each, where inſerted under the *Thorax,* is a hard protuberant conical Caſe or Shell, and ſomewhat in the Shape of a Muſcle-Shell, as will better be underſtood by viewing the Parts, B B B B, &c.

The Middle of the *Thorax* riſes very much at M, making a kind of blunt Cone, whereof M may be ſuppoſed the *Apex* About which greater Cone of the Body, the

ſmaller

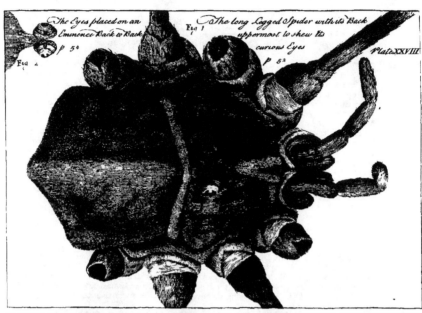

The Eyes placed on an
Emmence Back to Back
p 54

Fig 2

Fig 1

The long Legged Spider with its Back
uppermost to shew its
curious Eyes
p 52

Plate XXVIII

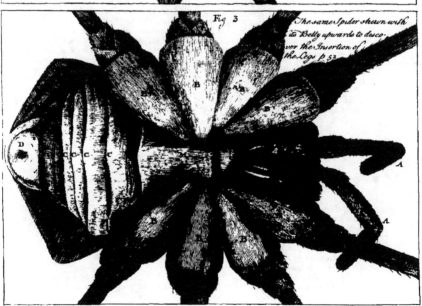

Fig 3

The same Spider shewn with
its Belly upwards to discover the Insertion of
the Legs p 52

ſmaller Cones of the Legs are placed, and extended almoſt to its Top, in ſuch a wonderful manner, as does not a little manifeſt the Wiſdom that contrived them ſo   For
theſe long Levers the Legs having no counter-acting long Body on the contrary Side of
the Centers whereon they move, muſt neceſſarily require a vaſt Strength to give them
Motion, and keep the Body ballanced and ſuſpended : inſomuch that if a Man's Body
were to be ſuſpended by ſuch a Contrivance, an hundred and fifty times the Strength of a
Man would be unſufficient to ſupport it and keep it from falling   To ſupply theſe Legs,
therefore, with proper Strength, each is furniſhed with a large ſhelly Caſe, which includes a very large and ſtrong Muſcle, whereby this little Creature is enabled, not only to
ſuſpend its Body on two or three of its Legs, but to move it very ſwiftly over the Tops of
Graſs and Leaves.

Beſides its eight Legs, this, like all other Sorts of Spiders, has two very ſhort Limbs
coming out before, which may be called its Arms, ſince the Uſe of them is not for walking, but to hold and turn its Prey. Each of theſe has three ſhort Joints, is thickly
covered with Hairs, and commonly appears bending as in the Figure A A

The Picture ſhews us likewiſe two double Claws K K in the Fore-part of its Head,
reſembling very much thoſe of a Scorpion, but differing a great deal from the Pincers or
Claws in moſt Kinds of Spiders, which ſtand horizontally, and ſerve to ſeize and wound
their Prey, and which when not made uſe of, are concealed in two Caſes contrived for
their Reception, whereinto they fold like a Claſp-Knife, and lie between a double Row of
Teeth.   Theſe Claws before us are undoubtedly for the ſame purpoſe, though particularly
adapted to the Manner of this Creature's taking its Prey, which it does by throwing its
Body at once upon it, inſtead of catching it with its Arms.

C C C C C, are certain Foldings in the Belly or Tail-Part of the Spider.   Thoſe on
the upper Side are all covered and defended by a ſtrong Shell, as may be ſeen in the firſt
Figure.

D, the Anus, whence little round Fæces or Pellets are excluded.

There are many Species of Spiders varying from one another in Size, Colour, Figure,
Way of Living, and many other Particularities, which would be tedious and improper to
mention in this Place, but the *Hunting-Spider* is ſo extraordinary, that ſome little Deſcription of it, with an Account of Mr. EVELYN's Obſervations on its Cunning and Dexterity, may, 'tis hoped, at leaſt not diſoblige the curious Reader.

Hunting-Spider

IT is a ſmall grey Spider, with Spots of Black over its whole Body, which are found by
the Microſcope to be made up of Feathers like thoſe on the Wings of Butterflies · Its
Motion is very nimble, ſometimes running, leaping at other times almoſt like a Graſhop-
per, then ſtopping ſhort, turning round on its hinder Legs with great Agility, and ſeeming to face every way   It has ſix Eyes, two in Front, looking directly forwards, two by
the Sides of theſe, pointing both forward and ſideways, and two others on the Middle of
its Back, which are the largeſt of all, and look backwards and ſideways   They are all
black, ſpherical, and finely poliſhed.

Theſe Spiders are a Sort of *Lupi*, which ſpin little or no Webs, but find a Harbour in
Chinks and Crevices of Walls and Houſes.   Mr. EVELYN ſays, he frequently obſerved
ſome of them at *Rome*, which eſpying a Fly, at three or four Yards Diſtance, upon the
Balcony where he ſtood, would not make directly to her, but crawl underneath the Rail,
till being got exactly againſt her, it would ſteal up, and ſpringing on her, ſeldom miſs its
Aim.   But if it chanced to want any thing of being directly oppoſite to the Fly, after
having peeped, it would immediately ſlink down again, and taking better Notice, would
come the next time directly on the Fly's Back   But if the Fly happened not to be within
its Leap, the Spider would move towards her ſo ſoftly, that the Motion of the Shadow
on a Dial is ſcarcely more imperceptible   However, if the Fly moved, the Spider would
move alſo in the ſame proportion, either forwards, backwards, or on either ſide, like a
well-managed Horſe, without turning its Body at all, keeping the ſame juſt Time with
the Fly's Motion as if the ſame Soul animated the Bodies of them both   But if the ca-
pricious Fly took Wing, and pitched upon ſome other Place behind the Spider, it would
whirl its Body round with all imaginable Swiftneſs, pointing its Head always towards the
Fly, tho' ſeemingly as immoveable, as if it had been a Nail driven into the Wood   Being got within a due Diſtance, by ſuch undiſcernable Approaches, it would then make a
Leap, ſwift as Lightning, upon the Fly, and catching him by the Pole, never afterwards
quit its hold till its Belly was quite full, when it would carry the Remainder home

He has likewife feen them inftructing their young ones how to hunt, and correcting them for Non-obfervance : And when any of the old ones chanced to mifs a Leap, they would run away, as if afhamed, into their Crannies, and not come out again for four or five Hours

Thefe Spiders are to be found with us on Garden-Walls, in the Spring, when the Weather is very hot, but they are not near fo eager of hunting as they are in *Italy*.

All Spiders are Creatures of Prey, though they have different Ways of catching it, fome by leaping, as the Sort juft now defcribed ; others by running on it as the *Shepherd-Spider* , but the greateft Number, by weaving Nets or Cob-webs, wherein they lie in Ambufh till Flies or other Infects are entangled, and then rufh out and feize them.

Spiders that make Webs have five little Teats or Nipples near the Extremity of the Tail, from whence a gummy Liquor iffues, which adheres to any thing it is preffed againft, and being drawn out, hardens inftantly in the Air, becoming a String or Thread ftrong enough to bear five or fix times the Weight of the Spider's Body, and yet of an amazing Finenefs.

They all lay Eggs, depofited in Bags, which they brood over, and guard with the utmoft Solicitude, and run away with at any Approach of Danger *. The Bags of fome are round white Balls carried under their Bellies , thofe of others appear like a little leathern Cap, faftned to a Leaf, or againft a Wall : Others again have two Bags of a reddifh Colour fufpended in fome Cranny by a Couple of Threads, with dry Leaves properly difpofed to fhelter them , and there are ftill other Varieties.

When hatched, the *little Spiders* come out compleatly formed, and run about very nimbly , fome Kinds being then exceeding hairy, and others perfectly fmooth They fhed their Skins feveral times, and increafe in Size, but never change their Shape at all.

An EXPLANATION of the TWENTY-NINTH PLATE.

The Ant, Emmet, or Pifmire.

Ant

THE Ant here delineated was of a large Kind, more than half the Bignefs of an Earwig, of a dark-brown or reddifh Colour, and extremely nimble A numerous Colony of them was difcovered under the Root of a Tree, whence they would frequently fally out in large Parties, and after doing much Mifchief amongft the Fruits and Flowers, and foraging over the whole Garden, would very readily find their Way back to the Neft again.

This Infect is naturally divided into the Head-Part, the Thorax or Breaft, and the Belly or Tail , each of which joins to the other by a very flender Ligament.

A A, The Ant's large Head , in which appear a Couple of globular and prominent black Eyes, moft curioufly pearled, B B Out of the Nofe or Snout iffue two pretty Horns C C, each having twelve Joints.

Its Jaws are Saw-like or indented, with little Teeth that exactly tally, opening fideways, and capable of gaping very wide afunder, D D. By the Help of thefe it is frequently feen grafping and tranfporting Bodies of three or four times its own Bulk and Weight

The Thorax feemed to confift of three rifing Parts E F G, and from thefe Parts three Legs, O O O, &c. fhaped like the Legs of a Fly, come forth on either fide

The Belly or Tail-Part, I I I, was larger than the other two, and joined to the Thorax by a very fmall conical Veftel H, which feemed a diftinct Part of the Animal, like a kind of loofe Shell interpofed to keep the Thorax from the Belly.

Two Circles of a lighter Colour went round the Tail-Part, as fhewn K K

There are feveral Species of Ants, differing both in Size and Colour : This given by the Doctor feems to be the large Wood-Ant Towards the End of Summer many of them are feen having four Wings. Thofe SWAMMERDAM fays, are Males

The

* *Memoires de l'Acad. des Scien Mr. de Reaumur,* 1710

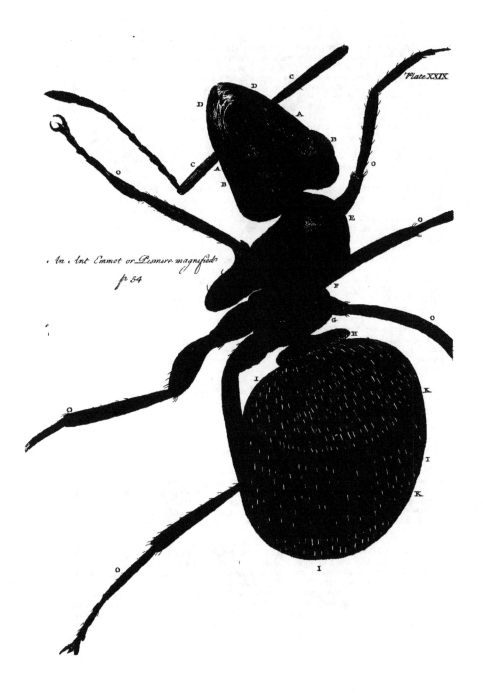

Plate XXIX

An Ant Emmet or Pismire magnified
p 54

The Tail of these Creatures is armed with a Sting, which they use however only when provoked, but then a poisonous Liquor is conveyed into the Wound, occasioning Pain and Swelling. The whole Body is cased over with a kind of Armour, so hard as scarce to be penetrated by a Lancet, thick-set with Multitudes of small white shining Bristles, the Legs, Horns, Head, &c are also full of Hairs, but smaller and darker.

This Kind of Ant, our Author says, would stand up on its hinder Legs, and raise its Head as high as possible, in order seemingly to enable it to see the farther.-----And putting his Finger towards them, they at first would all run to within a little Distance of it, where they would stand round at Bay, and smell, and consider, as it were, whether any of them should proceed farther; till one more daring than the rest venturing to climb it, all the others would have followed immediately, had he not prevented them. They are strong, vigorous, indefatigable, and very tenacious of Life, for a Trial of which one of them was put into Spirit of Wine, where after struggling for a pretty while, some Bubbles issued from its Mouth, and it remained quite motionless. It was left notwithstanding for above an Hour in the Spirit, when being taken out it seemed dead for about another Hour, but then on a sudden, like one that wakes out of a drunken Sleep, it revived and ran away. It was plunged again in the Spirit of Wine, where all the same Appearances were repeated, and on being taken out, after some time it came to Life in the same manner as before. On this it was the third time immerged in the same Liquor, (which is almost instant Death to most other Insects) and suffered to lie therein some Hours. But, notwithstanding, when it was taken out again, and had lain in a dry Place for three or four Hours, it recovered Life and Motion.

Ants live together in Colonies like Bees, and seem to have amongst them the same Kind of regular Government and Order. They have been famous in all Ages for their Industry in Summer, and their provident Care to lay up Stores of Sustenance against the Winter Season. There are none idle among them, but all of them are continually employed for the Utility of the Commonwealth. + We shall see one loaded with the Kernel of some Fruit, another bending beneath the Weight of a dead Gnat, and sometimes several together labouring to drag along the Carcass of some larger Insect. What can't be removed they eat upon the Spot, and thereby save so much of their own Stores, but carry home all that is capable of being preserved.

The whole Colony is not permitted to make Excursions at random. Some are detached as Scouts to gain Intelligence, and according to the Tidings they bring, all the Community are upon the March, which, as well as their Return, is under certain Regulations.

All the Ancients mention their amassing Stores of Corn and other Grain that will keep, and their gnawing away the Germen of every Grain, to prevent its shooting up; and indeed we shall see sometimes Ants carrying or pushing before them Grains of Wheat or Barley much larger than themselves. ALDROVANDUS also assures us, that he has seen their Granary, but as many of the Moderns, after diligent Search, have been unable to discover it, we have some reason to apprehend there may possibly be a Mistake as to this Particular, and that the Nymphæ which they often run about with in their Mouths, and which are sometimes of a yellow Colour, may have been taken for Corn without Buds, and swelled out by Moisture.

During the Winter-Season they conceal themselves in their Burrows under ground, where 'tis probable they lie torpid or buried in Sleep, like Multitudes of other Insects, and consequently eat very little. Their Industry, therefore, in storing up Provisions, is not so much intended to guard against the Winter, as to supply their young ones during the Harvest with necessary Sustenance. For they are regarded as Children of the State, and nourished as soon as they leave the Egg with an Assiduity that employs the whole Nation.

The Eggs of an Ant are of an oblong oval Figure, about the Size of Grains of Sand. From these little Worms are hatched, which after receiving their Food brought to them in common, and distributed in equal Proportions, leave off eating, wrap themselves up in a white Web, and sometimes in one that is yellow, and become Aureliæ, under which Form many People fancy they are the Eggs of Ants.

Whilst in the Aurelia State, they are guarded with the utmost Care, and removed from time to time, as the Circumstances of Things require. For the Ants either raise them towards the Surface of the Earth, or sink them to a Distance from it, as the Season is warm or cold, rainy or dry

+ Spectacle de la Nat. Dial. VIII.

'Tis

'Tis with incredible Care and natural Affection, says SWAMMERDAM, that Ants nourish and defend their *Aureliæ*, carrying them almost conftantly about with them in their Mouths, left any Mifchief fhould happen to them. He tells us, that keeping fome of them with their young ones in his Study, inclofed in a Glafs-Veffel filled with Earth, he obferved, with great Delight, that as the Superficies of the Earth grew dry, they carried their young ones deeper. And when he poured on fome Water, 'twas amazing to behold with how much Affection, Solicitude, and Eagernefs, they employed their utmoft Endeavours to remove them to fome fafer and drier Place. He often faw, after they had wanted Water for fome Days, that upon wetting the Earth a little, they would bring their young ones to that Place, where he could diftinctly fee them move and fuck in the Moifture. He tried frequently to bring up fome *Aureliæ* himfelf, but was always unfuccefsful, for though he took them when full of Nourifhment, no artificial Heat he could contrive was capable of making them come forth without the Affiftance of the Ants themfelves

Sir EDWARD KING, who was very curious in examining the Generation of thefe Creatures, obferves *, that in a Summer-Morning they bring up their *Aureliæ* towards the Top of the Bank, fo that from Ten o' Clock till Five or Six in the Afternoon, you may find them near the Top, and commonly on the South-fide But towards Seven or Eight at Night, if it be cool, or likely to rain, you may dig a Foot before you come at them †.

But nothing can be a ftronger Proof of the paternal Affection of thefe Creatures towards their Young, than what is fo very common that there are few People of the leaft Obfervation who have not feen it with their own Eyes : What I mean is, their running away with them in their Mouths whenever their Burrows are dug up or difturbed, bearing even Blows, and lofing their own Lives, rather than they will leave them in any Danger.

✤✤✤

An EXPLANATION of the THIRTIETH PLATE.

FIG. 1.

The Wandering Mite.

THE little Animal prefented to us in this Picture is called by Dr HOOKE, who was the firft Difcoverer of it, by the Name of the *Wandering Mite*, from its Likenefs both in Size and Shape to that very minute Infect. In *September* and *October* 1661, he perceived feveral of this Species wandering too and fro over the Glafs-Squares of his Chamber-Window at *Oxford*, and in the fame Months of the Year 1663, he obferved many of the fame Creatures creeping on a Glafs-Window at *London*, and examining the fubjacent Wall without the Window, he found Multitudes of them there alfo, running about among fome fmall Tufts of green Mofs, as well as amongft a curious blue and yellow minute Species of *Mufhroom*, or *Jews-Ear*, which grew upon the Wall.

This Creature appeared to the naked Eye to be a fort of black Mite, tho' nimbler and ftronger much than thofe found in Cheefe, but when viewed by the Microfcope, it was found to be finely crufted, or, as it were, cafed over with Armour.

The Belly Part A, which was very large in proportion to the reft of the Animal, feemed a protuberant oval Shell, thickly pitted with fmall Hollows, and covered all over with little white Briftles, whofe Points were directed backwards

The Middle-Part or *Thorax* was extremely fmall in Comparifon either of the Head or Belly, being only what we fee covered by the two Shells B B, though fpreading fomewhat larger underneath --- It is wonderful to confider with what Variety Nature proportions the Head, Thorax, and Belly of different Animals, in a manner unaccountable to us, but doubtlefs exactly fuited to the Way of Living and Happinefs of every diftinct Species

* *Vid Phil. Tranf* N° 23   † *Swammerd Bibl ad Hift Infect* p 153

I   The

The Head was shaped somewhat like a Mite's, having a long Snout in the manner of a Hog's, with a knobbed Ridge along the Middle of it, C. This Ridge was befet on both fides with many fmall Briftles all pointing forwards. Two very large and long Briftles or Horns, D D, proceeded alfo from the Top of the Head, juft above the Eyes, and pointed the fame way

Its Legs were eight in Number, iffuing from the Thorax, and each of them armed with a very fharp Talon or Claw at its Extremity, which in walking faftned into the Pores of any Body it went over. Thefe Legs were furnifhed at every Joint with great Numbers of fmall Hairs, all directed and pointing towards the Claws.

Our Author tells us, that by finding thefe Infects, he apprehended he had difcovered the Vagabond Parents of fuch Mites as we meet with on Cheefes, Meal, Corn, Seeds, mufty Barrels, mufty Leather, and many other Bodies, which little Creatures wandering about at random, and finding an agreeable Pafture, might fpend their Lives and leave a plentiful Offspring behind them on different putrid Subftances, and that the new Generations, by fuch Alteration in their Habitation and Diet, may, like Colonies brought from the Southern into the Northern Countries, or *vice verfa*, after fome Defcents, change both their Shape and Colour.

We leave the Probability of this Suppofition to be confidered by the Curious, who will better be enabled to pafs their Judgment, by comparing this Figure with that of the *Cheefe-Mite*, which is given in the next Plate

PLATE XXX. FIG. 2.

The Crab-like Infect.

D R HOOKE informs us, that obferving, one Day in *September*, a very fmall Infect creeping flowly over a Book he was reading, he placed it before his Microfcope, and found its Form fo unufual that he made a Drawing of it.

Its Size was about the Bignefs of a large Mite, but fomewhat longer It had ten Legs, eight whereof, *a a a a a a a a*, terminated with exceeding fharp Claws, and were thofe upon which it walked They appeared much like the fmall Legs of a Crab, both as to their Hairinefs and the Number of their Joints, and this Infect refembled a Crab in many other Particulars For the two foremoft and largeft Legs B B, which appeared to grow from the Head, where the Horns of other Animals come out, were formed exactly in the manner of a Crabs larger Claws, being fhaped and jointed as in the Picture, and furnifhed with Pincers C C, which the Animal opened and fhut at pleafure It feemed to employ thefe two Horns or Claws both as Feelers and Holders, for in its Walking it carried them aloft and extended forward, moving them too and fro, as a Man blind folded would do his Hands to feel out his Way before him, and if a Hair was put to them, they would readily catch hold of it, and feem to hold it faft

D D were two black Spots, which, by their Form and the bright Reflections from them, feemed to be the Eyes

E E, two Pair of Forceps placed near its Mouth, in Readinefs to catch or hold its Prey, and convey it thither

The whole Infect was cafed over with fhelly Coverings, like other cruftaceous Animals The Head F appeared a kind of fcaly Shell, and ended in a fharp Snout like that of a Lobfter The Thorax G G confifted of two fmooth circular Shells or Rings, and the Belly of eight more, thickly covered with little Knobs or Protuberancies.

Whether any Wings were concealed under thefe laft Shells could no way be difcovered, but from its Number of Legs the contrary is moft probable; for fcarce any winged Infect is found with eight Legs, whereas fuch whofe Legs are no more than fix, are ufually fupplied with Wings

This Infect is rarely found.

Q

PLATE

PLATE XXX. FIG. 3.

Cloth-Worm, or Moth.

Cloth Worm   THIS pretty Infect is the *Tinea Argentea*, or *Cloaths-Moth* in its Worm-State, tho' called the *Book Worm* by Dr HOOKE, from his having often feen it running amongft Books and Papers. It is of a white-fhining Silver or Pearl-Colour, is commonly found lurking in Holes or Crannies, and whenever it is difturbed, fcuds away very nimbly to feek fome other Hiding-Place

The Head-Part to the naked Eye appears with a blunt End, with a Body growing fmaller and fmaller, and tapering towards the Tail, but when the Microfcope is employed, the little blunt Head of this Infect is found furnifhed on either fide with a Clufter of pearled Eyes, though the Pearls are fewer than in other Infects whofe Eyes are thus conftructed Each Eye is furrounded with a Row of fmall Hairs, much like the *Cilia* or Hairs of the Eyelids, and perhaps may ferve for the fame purpofe It has two long ftrait Horns, A A, tapering towards the Top, moft curioufly jointed, with Rings or Circles of Hairs iffuing from and encompaffing each Joint, and feveral larger Briftles interfperfed here and there amongft them. Befides thefe, it has alfo two fhorter Horns or Feelers B B, jointed and incircled with Hairs like the former, but without any Briftles, and ending with blunted Points.

The conical Body of this Creature confifts of fourteen feveral Shells or Shields, folding over each other like jointed Pieces of Armour, and covering the whole Body, and each of thefe is again tiled over, as it were, with a Multitude of thin tranfparent Scales, which, from the great Number of their reflecting Surfaces, make the whole Animal appear of a Pearl-Colour. Its Sides are armed with many long, fharp and ftrong Briftles From the hinder Part three Tails proceed, C C C, refembling in all refpects, the two longer Horns growing from the Head.

Notwithftanding the Suppofition of our Author, that this Creature feeds upon Papers and the Covers of Books, and makes the Holes that are oftentimes found therein, Mr. ALBIN afferts it to be the very Animal that eats Cloths or Stuffs made of Woollen; and fays, it is produced from a fmall grey fpeckled Moth, that flies about in the Night, creeps in among woollen Things, and there lays her Eggs, which after a time are hatched by the natural Heat of the Woollen, and the little Blood feed thereon till they change into flying Moths like their Parent.

As for the Holes in Books and Papers, they are probably made by the fame little nimble minute Infect which eats Holes of a like Size and Form in Picture-Frames, Chair-Frames, and other Things made of Wood, and which, from its Refemblance in Shape and Bignefs is called the little *Wood-Loufe*

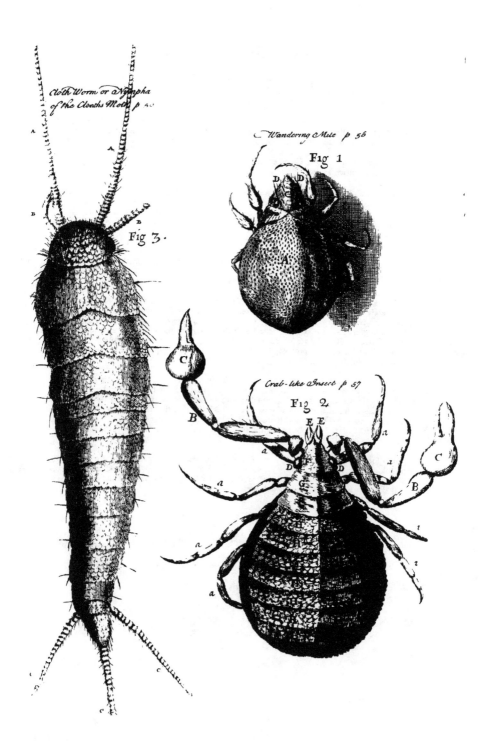

Cloth Worm or Nympha
of the Cloaths Moth p 50

Fig 3.

Wandering Mite p 56
Fig 1

Crab-like Insect p 57
Fig 2

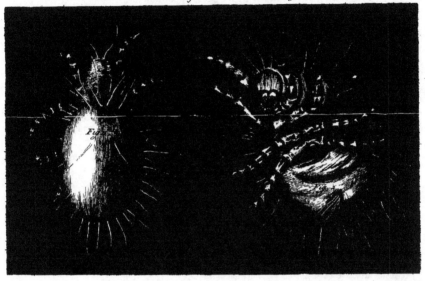

A Small Creature hatched on a Vine p 60

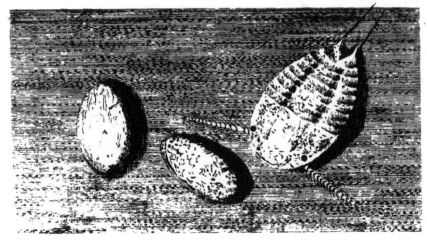

An EXPLANATION of the THIRTY-FIRST PLATE.

FIG. 1.

A Cheeſe-Mite with its Back uppermoſt.

THERE are ſeveral Species of minute Creatures, which from their extreme Small- Cheeſe-Mite
neſs and ſome Reſemblance in Form, are called by the general Name of *Mites*. One on its Belly
Sort of theſe was ſhewn and deſcribed in the *Plate* immediately preceding, and there
called the *Wandering-Mite*, from its being found abroad, and rambling as it were at
large.

The Figure under our Eye at preſent is one of the Mites found in Cheeſe, placed in a
crawling Poſture with the Back-Part uppermoſt   The Shape is a kind of Oval, but more
obtuſe at the Tail-End.   It has three Regions or Parts as in larger Inſects   The hinder
Part or Belly A ſeems covered with one intire Shell, ſo curiouſly poliſhed, that, as in a
convex Looking-Glaſs, it ſhews the Pictures of all the Objects round about.   The
Middle, or Cheſt, ſeems divided and covered with two Shells B C, which running
one within the other, the Mite is able to draw in or thruſt out as it finds Occaſion , and
it can do the ſame with its Snout D

The whole Body is cruſtaceous, of a Pearl-Colour, and pretty tranſparent, ſo that divers Motions of the Inteſtines may be diſcerned within it   Several long white Hairs grow
out from it in different Places, ſome of which are longer than the whole Animal, though
in the Drawing they are not ſo repreſented.   They all appear pretty ſtrait and pliable,
excepting two that iſſue from the Head-Part, and ſeem to be the Horns

PLATE XXXI. FIG. 2.

A Cheeſe-Mite with its Belly upwards.

THIS ſecond Figure ſhews a Mite that was ſomewhat larger than the former, fixed A Mite on it
on the Back-Part of its Tail, by means of a little *Mouth-Glew* rubbed on the Ob- B c
ject Plate, with Deſign to exhibit the Inſertion of the Legs, and ſuch other Particulars as
eſcaped the firſt Examination.

To the ſmall End of the oval Body the Head is faſtned, (very little in proportion to the
other Parts) where a Pair of Eyes may be diſtinguiſhed, appearing like two dark minute
Specks   The Mouth reſembles that of a Mole, opening and ſhutting occaſionally, and
when open appearing red within   It has little Briſtles at the Snout, and if one has the
good Luck to view it at a proper Time, one ſhall ſee it munching and chewing the Cud
like a *Guinea-Pig*

It is furniſhed with eight well-ſhaped and proportioned Legs covered with a very tranſparent Shell   Each Leg has eight Joints, fringed as it were with ſeveral ſmall Hairs   The
Struxture of the Joints ſeems the ſame as in the Legs of Crabs and Lobſters, and each Leg
is armed with a very ſharp Claw or Hook at its End, in the ſame manner as theirs are
Four of theſe Legs are ſo placed as to move the Body forwards   The other four, by being diſpoſed in a quite contrary Direction, draw it backwards when there is Occaſion

Mites appear to the naked Eye merely like Duſt in Motion , nor is the ſharpeſt Sight
able to diſtinguiſh their Parts, unleſs aſſiſted by Glaſſes   They are Male and Female
The Females lay Eggs, from which very ſmall Mites are hatched, of the ſame Shape with
their Parents   for theſe Creatures ſhed their Skins ſeveral times, and increaſe in Bigneſs, but
never change their Form.   A Mite's Egg is not more than a four or five hundredth Part
of the Size of a well-grown Mite , and ſuch Mites are not much above one hundredth
of an Inch in Thickneſs   So that, according to this Way of reckoning, no leſs than a
Million of full-grown Mites may be contained in a cubic Inch, and five times as many Eggs

The various Sorts of Mites, to be met with up and down in divers putrifying Subſtances,
are very different in Shape, Colour, Size, and ſeveral other Properties, according, perhaps,
to the Nature of the Subſtances whereon they are nouriſhed.   Thoſe found on ſome Bodies are longer, on others rounder, ſome more hairy, others ſmoother   In this nimble, in
that ſlow, here pale and whiter, there browner, blacker, more tranſparent, &c.   But
they all agree in being exceedingly voracious.

PLATE XXXI. FIG. 3.

A fmall Creature hatched on a Vine.

DURING moft part of the Spring and Summer, a fmall, round, white, Cobweb-like Subftance, about the Bignefs of a Pea, may be found fticking, very clofe and faft, to the Stocks of Vines nailed againft a warm Wall.

When examined attentively, it feems covered, on the upper Side, with a fmall Hufk, not unlike the Scale or Shell of the *Wood-Loufe*, *Millepes*, or *Sow*, (for by all thefe Names is the Infect called which is often found in rotten Wood, and on being touched rolls itfelf into the Size and Shape of a Pepper-Corn.) Several of thefe being feparated from the Vine-Stock, the Doctor found them, by his Microfcope, to confift of a Shell, which feemed likely to be the Hufk of a *Millipes*, and the Fur or Cobweb confifted of Abundance of fmall Filaments. He often difcovered in the Middle of all great Numbers of fmall brown Eggs, fuch as A and B reprefent. They were about the Bignefs of the Eggs of Mites, and were ufually hatched about the End of *June* or Beginning of *July*, produc-ing Multitudes of fmall Infects exactly fhaped like that marked *x*

The Head of this Creature was very large, being almoft half the Bignefs of its Body, as is ufual in the *Fœtus* of moft Animals It had two fmall black Eyes *a a*, and two long, flender, jointed and briftled Horns *b b*. The hinder Part of its Body feemed to con-fift of nine Scales, and the laft ended in a forky Tail, much like that of a Wood-Loufe, out of which iffued two long Hairs

They ran to and fro very brifkly, moft were about the Size of a common Mite, but others lefs. The longeft of them, however, feemed not the hundredth Part of an Inch, and the Eggs ufually not above half as much. They appeared to have fix Legs, though none are fhewn in the Picture, the Legs being commonly drawn under the Body, and al-moft hid thereby.

Our Author obferves, that if thefe little Creatures are *Wood-Lice*, (as he is inclined to think, from their Shape, Frame, and the Skin or Shell upon them) they afford an In-ftance of a furprifing and more than ordinary Increafe in Bignefs, from their prefent Mi-nutenefs when newly hatched, to the Size they attain when fully grown For a common *Wood Loufe* of half an Inch long, is no lefs than an hundred and twenty five thoufand times bigger than one of thefe ---Some Sorts of Spiders have alfo nearly the fame Propor-tion to their young ones when newly hatched.

What the Hufk and Cobweb of this little white Subftance fhould be, our Author can-not imagine, unlefs the old one, when impregnated with Eggs, fhould fix itfelf on the Vine and die there, after which its Body rotting away by degrees, nothing appears re-maining but the Hufk and Eggs only.

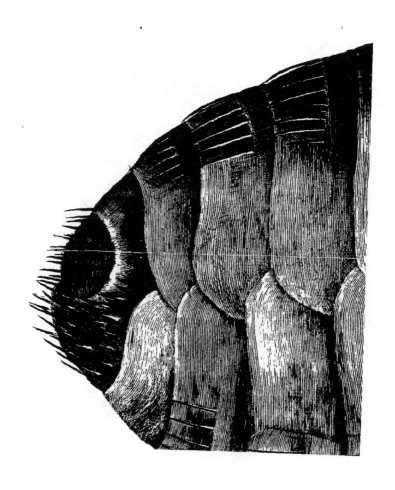

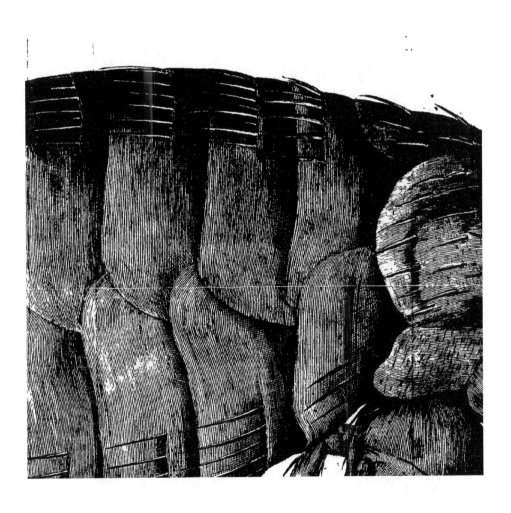

Plate XXXII

The FLEA

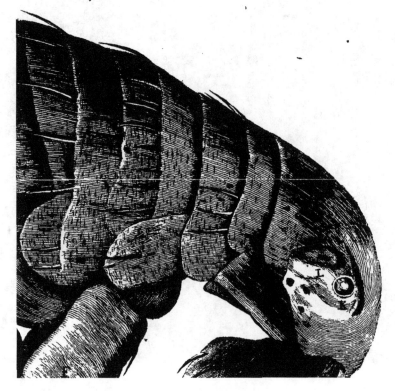

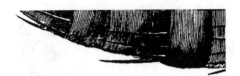

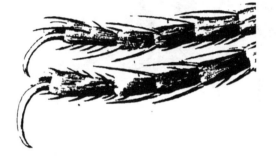

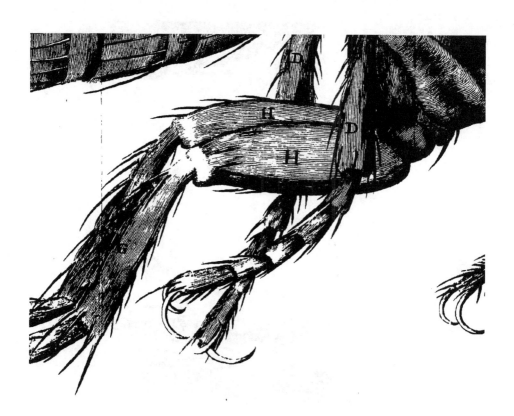

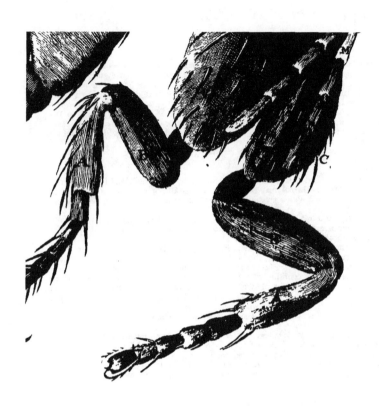

An EXPLANATION of the THIRTY-SECOND PLATE.

The Flea.

THOUGH this little Creature is almoſt univerſally known to be a ſmall brown *The Flea* ſkipping Animal, very few are acquainted with its real Shape and Figure, with the Structure, Strength and Beauty of its Limbs and Parts, or with the Manner of its Generation and Increaſe, Circumſtances which could never have been diſcovered but by the Aſſiſtance of the Microſcope.

The Body of this Creature is of an oval Form, compoſed of ſeveral ſhelly Scales or Diviſions moſt curiouſly jointed, and folding over one another, thoſe that cover the Back meeting thoſe that cover the Belly on each Side of the Body, and lying, alternately, over one and under another of them.

Its Neck is finely arched, and much reſembling a *Lobſter*'s Tail in Shape, moving too like that, very nimbly, by means of the joining and folding over of the Scales that cover it.

The Head is ſmall and ſhelly, having on each ſide a quick, round, and beautiful black Eye K, in the Middle whereof may be ſeen a round blackiſh Spot, which is the Pupil of the Eye ‡, encompaſſed with a greeniſh glittering Circle or *Iris*, as bright and vivid as the Eye of a Cat.

Behind each Eye a ſmall Cavity appears at L, wherein a certain thin Film, beſet with many ſmall tranſparent Hairs, may be obſerved moving to and fro, which our Author imagines may probably be the Ear.

From the Snout-Part proceed the two Fore-Legs, and between them are two long ſmall Feelers (or Smellers, as our Author ſuppoſes) M M Each of them has four Joints and Abundance of little Hairs. Juſt below and almoſt between theſe Horns, lies the *Proboſcis* or Peircer N N O, conſiſting of a Tube N N, and a Tongue or Sucker O, which can be put out or drawn in at pleaſure. It has alſo two Chaps or Biters P P, ſhaped ſomewhat like the Blades of a Pair of round-top'd Sciſſars, and ſeeming to open and ſhut after the ſame manner. The Flea with theſe Inſtruments penetrates the Skin of living Creatures, and leaves a round red Spot behind it, which we commonly term a *Flea-Bite*.

All the Shells and ſcaly Coverings of this pretty Inſect are moſt exquiſitely poliſhed, and in Colour reſembling fine Tortoiſe-Shell, the Scales on the Back and Belly have each of them along its Middle a Row of ſtrong ſharp Briſtles pointing towards the Tail, like the Quills of Porcupines, and as large as they in proportion to the Animal The Neck and Shoulders are likewiſe armed in the ſame manner, and great Numbers of Briſtles are placed about the Tail.

But the curious Structure and Contrivance of its Legs are more particularly deſerving our Examination and Praiſe, being ſuch as have not been diſcovered in any other Creature, and are adapted peculiarly to the Exigencies of this, for as it lives by ſucking human Blood, or the Blood of other living Animals, which cannot be obtained without inflicting Wounds and cauſing Pain, which muſt neceſſarily produce Reſentment, and a Deſire of Revenge, it was abſolutely requiſite the little Invader ſhould have ſome ready Means of Eſcape, ſince every Meal muſt otherwiſe be paid for with its Life. As therefore it has no Wings, its Safety muſt be entirely owing to its Legs, and indeed they are moſt excellently fitted for this purpoſe, by folding ſhort one within another, and then ſtretching out to their whole Length with a ſudden Spring or Jerk, whereby they commonly deliver the little Animal from the Danger of a Purſuit.

The Parts A A, of the Fore-Legs, lie within the Parts B B, and thoſe again within the upper and ſtronger Parts C C, parallel to, or ſide by ſide with each other But the Parts of the two next Legs are diſpoſed directly contrary to theſe; for in them the Parts D D are placed without the Parts E E, and the Parts E E are likewiſe more outward ſtill than the Parts F F In the hinder Legs the Parts G, H, and I, bend one within another, like the Limbs of a double-jointed Ruler, or like the Foot, Leg and Thigh of a Man When the Flea intends to leap, he folds up theſe ſix Legs together, then ſprings them all out at the ſame inſtant, and thereby exerting his whole Strength at once, carries his little Body to a conſiderable Diſtance. His Legs have three principal and larger ſtrong Parts, and below them many ſmall Joints or Diviſions as in the Legs of a Fly From every Joint proceed long Hairs or Briſtles, and each Foot is furniſhed with a Pair of long-hooked

R   Claw-

‡ Vid *Power*'s *Obſerv.* p. 1

Claws or Talons, that in his Leaping he may faften and cling the better to what he lights upon.

Fleas are produced of Eggs, which the Females ftick faft by a kind of glutinous Moi-fture to the Roots of the Hairs of Cats, Dogs, and other Animals, and alfo to the Wool in Blankets, Ruggs, and other fuch-like Furniture. Of thefe Eggs a Female lays ten or twelve a Day, for feveral Days fucceffively, and they hatch in the fame Order, about four or five Days after their being laid

From the Eggs come forth not perfect Fleas, but little whitifh Worms or Maggots, whofe Bodies have annular Divifions, and are thinly covered with long Hairs. They ad-here clofely to the Body of the Animal, on whofe Juices they feed, or they may be kept in a Box, and brought up with dead Flies, which they eat with Greedinefs They are very brifk and nimble, and crawl like Catterpillars, with a lively and brifk Motion.

After eleven Days from the Time of their being hatched, they forbear eating, and lie quiet, feemingly, as if dying, but if viewed with a Microfcope, they will be found weav-ing a Covering or Bag round them with a Silk or Web emitted out of their Mouth. In this Bag they put on the *Chryfalis* or *Aurelia* Form, and become milk-white They con-tinue nine Days under this Appearance, their Colour darkens by degrees, they acquire Firmnefs and Strength, and as foon as they iffue from the Bag are perfect Fleas, and able to leap away They are immediately capable of Coition, and lay Eggs in three or four Days, after which they foon die, as all other Creatures that undergo thefe Changes do.

The great Agility and Strength of this Infect are exceedingly remarkable, it being able to leap farther in proportion to its own Length, than perhaps any other Creature that has not Wings to help it And its Strength is fo well known, and fo extraordinary in the fame proportion, that feveral curious Artifts, whofe Dexterity has been fhewn in the making Curiofities of an uncommon and furprifing Smallnefs, have employed this little Animal to affift in exhibiting their Works, and proving the Nicety and Lightnefs of them Dr. POWER fays *, he faw amongft TREDESCANT's Rarities, a golden Chain of three hun-dred Links, though not above an Inch long, that was both faftened to and drawn away by a Flea MOUFFET fome time before this, mentions fuch another of a Finger's Length, made by one MARK an *Englifhman* †, whereto a Flea was faftned by a Collar of a moft exquifite Minutenefs, with a Lock and Key adapted to it This Chain the Flea dragged after him with Eafe, the Flea, Chain, Lock and Key, not exceeding altogether the Weight of a fingle Grain He adds further, that he had been informed by People of undoubted Credit, that a Coach made of Gold with all its Furniture of the fame Metal, had a Flea chained to it, which drew it along without the leaft Difficulty, thereby tefti-fying at the fame time the Dexterity of the Workman, and the Strength of this little Creature Nor is there any Room to doubt the Truth of thefe Accounts, for one Bo-VERICK, a Watchmaker in the *Strand*, has lately made and fhewn to vaft Numbers of People, not only a Chaife having four Wheels and all its proper Apparatus, together with a Man fitting therein, the whole formed of Ivory, and drawn along by a Flea, but likewife a *Landau* that opens and fhuts by Springs, with fix Horfes harnefs'd thereto, a Coachman fitting on the Box with a Dog between his Legs, four People in the *Landau*, two Foot-men behind it, and a Poftilion riding one of the Fore-Horfes This Equipage a Flea is faftned to, and pulls very eafily along. He has alfo made a Chain of Brafs, about two Inches in Length, containing two hundred Links, with a Hook at one End, and a Padlock and Key at the other, all which together weigh lefs than the third Part of a Grain. Here too a Flea is made ufe of to draw the Chain, which it does very nimbly, and with as little Trouble as can be well imagined.

Fleas thus employed are preferved alive and vigorous, by putting them upon the Arm, or the Back of the Hand to feed, once or twice a Day.

But however pretty they may be in the Microfcope, or for thefe ingenious Purpofes, they are certainly very troublefome Bedfellows, and efpecially to Women and Children, whofe Blood they are particularly fond of. They hide themfelves in the Woolinefs of the Blankets all the Day, but as foon as People begin to be warm in their Beds at Night, which they are fenfible of either by their Smell or fome other Way, they creep between the Sheets, and penetrating the moft tender Parts of the Body, fuck out the Blood and Humours They have likewife the Sagacity to retire at Day-break to their lurking Holes again, as if afraid of being caught And in this they are imitated by the *Punices* or *Bugs*, which

* *Power's Obferv* p 3   † *Moufet Infectorum Theatr* p 275

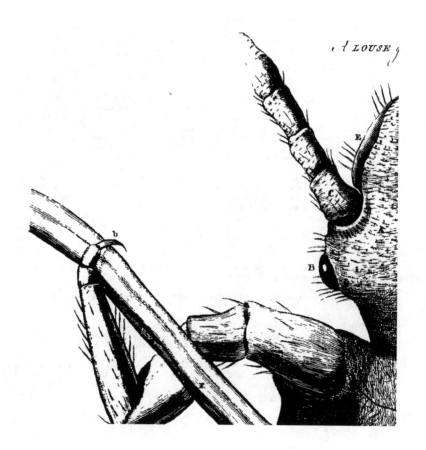

Plate XXXIII

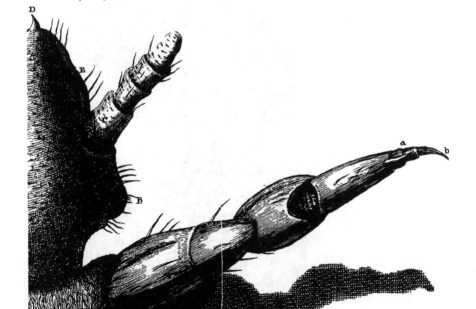

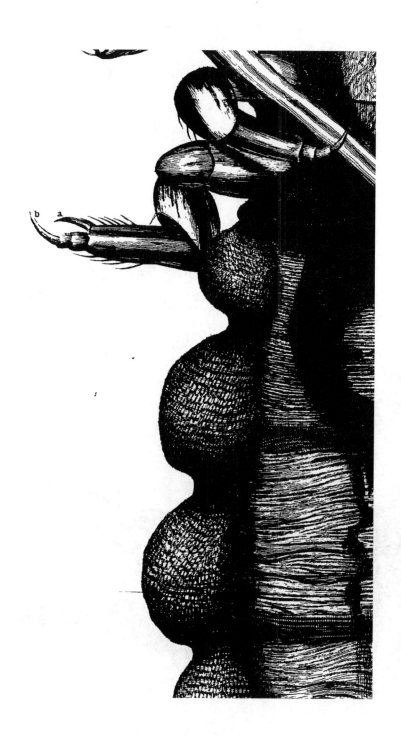

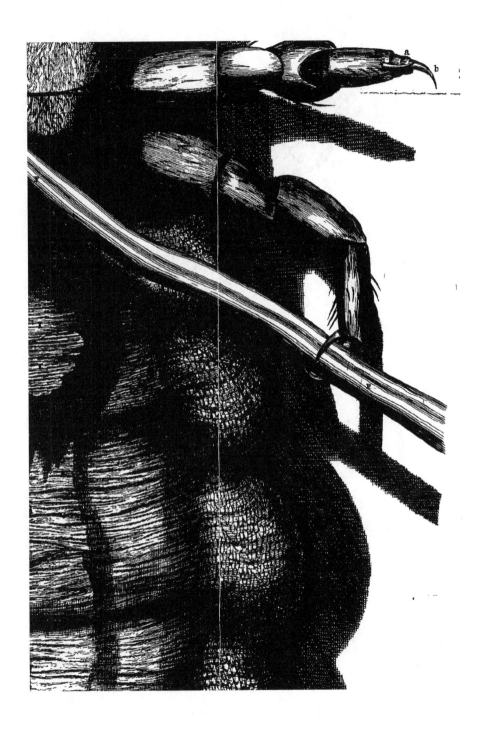

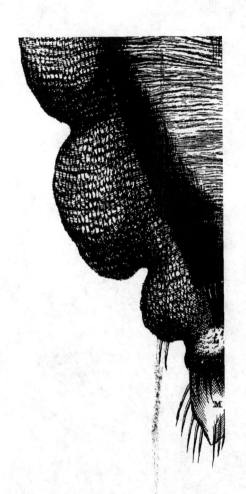

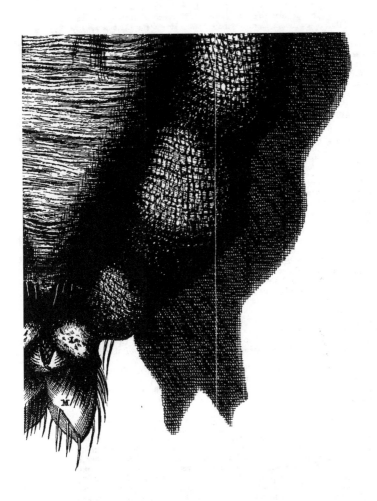

which are Animals much more nafty and mifchievous, having fomewhat poifonous in their Bite, as the Swelling that follows upon it fhews. The Smell of thefe is alfo extremely offenfive, and that as it fhould feem even to Fleas, for where there are many *Bugs* Fleas are but feldom feen.

Many Sorts of Herbs, if placed about the Bed, are faid to deftroy, or at leaft drive away Fleas, fuch as *Elder, Fern, Penny-Royal, Rue, Mint, Hops, Laurel, Walnut, Arfmart, Hellebore,* &c alfo the Seeds of *Staves-Acre, Coriander, Flea-Wort,* &c. but without doubt the moft effectual Remedy is Cleanlinefs

If you attempt to catch them, remember always to wet your Thumb and Finger with Spittle

An Explanation of the Thirty-Third Plate.

The Loufe.

THIS laft Plate fhews us the Figure of a Loufe magnified to a very great Degree, that every Part thereof may be perfectly known and diftinguifhed : And indeed this Creature is fo tranfparent, that the internal Structure, Difpofition, and Motion of its Bowels, and their Contents, may be difcerned therein much better than they can in moft other Infects. *The Loufe*

It is reprefented in this Picture with its Belly upwards, grafping a Hair between its Claws.

The Head A, fomewhat refembles the Fafhion of a Cone, but is a little flatted on the upper and under Part. On each Side, juft where the Head is wideft, a large fhining black Eye appears, very protuberant, and encompaffed with a Number of fmall Hairs Thefe Eyes B B, are fituated a little behind the Head, in the Place where the Ears of other Creatures ftand, and where one would expect to find the Eyes, a Couple of Horns come out C C, extending themfelves in fuch a manner, that they defend its Eyes from being injured by the Hairs through which it paffes.

Our Author fays, each of thefe Horns has four Joints, fringed as it were with fmall Briftles, and the Picture C C fhews no more than that Number of Divifions, but Swammerdam reckons five Joints to each Horn of the Loufe he defcribes * ; fo that either the Lice thefe two Obfervers examined, were of a different Species, or one of them muft be miftaken.

The Head grows round and tapering from where the Horns come out to the Top of the Snout D, which ends in a fharp Point, and feems to be a tubular Inftrument whereby the Loufe fucks in the Blood of the Animal it feeds on, it is likewife probably the Sheath of a Peircer that ferves to penetrate the Skin and make a Wound for the Blood to iffue out

In the Pofition before us, there feems to be a Refemblance of Chaps or Jaws, as at the Letters E E, yet when placed in another View thofe Lines or Appearances are not difcernable. Swammerdam fays, it has no Mouth that opens ; and our Author obferves, that having kept feveral of them in a Box for two or three Days, whereby they were become extremely hungry, upon letting one creep on his Hand, he found that it immediately fell to Sucking, and though it neither feemed to thruft its Nofe very deep into the Skin, nor to open any kind of Mouth, he could plainly difcern a fmall Current of Blood paffing directly fiom its Snout into its Belly, and there appeared about A fome Contrivance like a Pump, Pair of Bellows, or Heart, which by a very fwift and alternate Dilatation and Contraction drew up the Blood from the Nofe and forced it into the Body Though he viewed it very attentively while fucking, he could not perceive that any more of its Nofe was thruft into the Skin than the very Snout D; nor did it give him the leaft Pain, notwithftanding the Blood ran through its Head very quick and freely. Which fully proves that Blood-Veffels are difperfed into every Part of the *Skin*, nay, even into the *Cuticula*, for had its whole Snout been thruft in from D to C C, it would not have amounted to the fuppofed Thicknefs of that Tegument, the Length of the whole Nofe not being more than the three hundredth Part of an Inch

The Thorax or Breaft is covered with a thin, tranfparent, horny, or fhelly Subftance, which did not fink or become fhrivelled by the Creature's fafting, as the Covering of the Belly did. Through this our Author could plainly diftinguifh that the Blood fucked from his

I   * *Swammerd Hift Gener, des Infect.* p 174

Obſervations on the Louſe.

his Hand was variouſly diſtributed and moved to and fro, and about G there appeared a pretty large white Subſtance moving within the *Thorax*. This ſomewhat reſembled a Bladder, contracting and dilating upwards and downwards from the Head towards the Tail. Acroſs the Breaſt were many ſmall milk-white Veſſels running between the Legs, and ſending to them innumerable minute Branchings, which no doubt are Veins and Arteries; for in moſt Inſects the Juices analogous to Blood are white.

The Louſe has ſix Legs, which are ſtrongly joined to the *Thorax*, and for each Pair a kind of Diviſion appears thereon, as *e e e* They are covered with a very tranſparent Shell, and jointed exactly like the Legs of a Crab or Lobſter Each of them is divided into ſix Parts, having ſeveral ſmall Hairs iſſuing therefrom, and Ends with two Claws, of unequal Lengths, very properly adapted to the particular Exigences of this Animal, which has Occaſion to walk either on Skin or Hair For the leſſer Claw *a* being ſo much ſhorter than the other Claw *b*, when it walks on Skin the ſhorter Claw touches not, and then the Feet are the ſame as thoſe of a *Mite* and many other Inſects: Whereas, when amongſt Hairs, the longer Claw can bend itſelf round by means of its ſmall Joints, and meeting with the ſhorter, can both together take hold and graſp a Hair, as with a Thumb and Finger, after the manner repreſented in the Figure, where F F F, the Hair of a Man's Head, is ſo graſped and held faſt by this Creature, that it is in no danger of falling from it

The Belly is likewiſe very tranſparent, but its Covering bears the Reſemblance of a Skin rather than a Shell, being grained all over juſt like the Skin of a Man's Hand, and when the Belly is empty, growing very flaccid and wrinkled

H H ſhew the Stomach placed in the upper Part of the Belly.

The white Spot I I, may poſſibly be the *Liver* or *Pancreas*, which, by the *periſtaltic* Motion of the Guts, is moved a little to and fro, not with a *Syſtole* and *Diaſtole*, but rather with a thronging or juſtling Motion.

After one of theſe Creatures had faſted two Days, all the hinder Parts appeared lank and wrinkled; the white Subſtance I I, ſcarcely moved, moſt of the white Branchings diſappeared, as did alſo the Redneſs or ſucked Blood in the Guts, the *periſtaltic* Motion whereof was hardly to be diſcerned, but upon ſuffering it to ſuck, the Skin of the Belly, and the ſix ſcalloped Emboſſments on either ſide, were quickly filled out, the Stomach and Guts ſeemed quite crammed, and Multitudes of white Veſſels appeared replete and turgid, the *periſtaltic* Motion grew quick, and ſo did alſo the juſtling Motion of the Subſtance I I

The Animal was ſo voracious, that notwithſtanding it could contain no more, it continued ſucking as greedily as ever, and at the ſame time emptied itſelf as faſt behind. And its Digeſtion muſt needs be very quick, for though the Blood, when ſucked, appeared thin and black, it ſoon became in the Guts of a lovely Ruby-colour, and that Part of it which was carried into the Veins was evidently white: Whereby we alſo find, that a further Digeſtion of Blood may make it Milk, or at leaſt of a milky Colour.

Near the Bottom of the Belly appears the Anus K, beſet with Hairs or Briſtles, juſt below are two little Parts L L, ſomewhat of a ſemicircular Figure, whoſe Inſides are covered with a Down, and which ſerve, occaſionally, to cover and cloſe the Aperture of the Anus At the Extremity of the Tail are a Couple of Bodies M M, reſembling the Rumps of Fowls, from whence iſſue a Number of ſharp Hairs.

Dr POWER takes notice, that having placed a Louſe on its Back, in the Poſition here before us, there were two bloody darkiſh Spots diſcernable, the greater in the Midſt of the Body, and the leſſer towards the Tail In the Center of the larger Spot there is (ſays he) a white Film or Bladder, which continually contracts and dilates itſelf upwards and downwards, and always, after every Pulſe of this white Particle or Veſicle, there follows a Pulſe of the great dark bloody Spot, in which, or over which this Veſicle ſeems to ſwim This he obſerved two or three Hours together, as long as the Louſe lived, for pricking the white Veſicle with a ſmall Needle, which let out a ſmall Drop of Blood, and then viewing it again with the *Microſcope*, no Signs of Life or Motion could be perceived.

Lice proceed from Parents of their own Kind, and not (as formerly was ſuppoſed) from certain Juices or Humours of human Bodies, which may ſerve indeed to nouriſh, but can never breed them The Females lay Eggs, or Nits, which they faſten to the Hair of the Head, or to other hairy or woolly Subſtances, by a glewy Matter wherewith

they

they are provided. From theſe, *young Lice* come forth perfect in all their Members, and
undergo no other Change but an Increaſe of Size

Mr. LEEUWENHOEK diſcovered, that the Males are armed with Stings in their Tails,
which the Females have not, and as he felt little or no Pain from ſeven or eight Lice
that were feeding on his Hand at once, he imagines the ſmarting Pain they ſometimes
give muſt ariſe from their Stinging, when made uneaſy by Preſſure or otherwiſe, for if
roughly treated, they may be ſeen to thruſt out their Stings

MOUFET † makes a Difference between the Lice of the Body and thoſe of the Head
The latter (he tells us) are larger, longer, flatter, and more nimble, the former fatter,
rounder belly'd, ſlower, and of a whiter Colour, with ſome blackiſh Lines or Streaks.
He alſo informs us, that if Lice are rubbed gently between the Thumb and Finger, they
feel as if they were ſquare, and ſomewhat harder than Fleas, from which, by ſo doing,
they may be diſtinguiſhed even in the dark.

Having now deſcribed and explained all the Plates Dr HOOKE has left
of Objects examined by the Microſcope, with ſuch Brevity and Plain-
neſs, as may, 'tis hoped, be uſeful and agreeable ; and added thereto
many Obſervations on the *Subjects* he has laid before us, in order to
make this Work more valuable: We ſhall take leave of the *Reader*,
with this ſingle, but neceſſary Reflection: That whenever we behold,
in any of the Operations of Nature, whether great or ſmall, a *Contrivance*, a *Regularity*, a *Beauty*, that both delights and ſurprizes,
we ſhould not paſs it over without Conſideration as a Matter of mere
Amuſement, but take Occaſion from thence, to raiſe our Thoughts
from the *Creature* to the *Creator*, and therein contemplate and adore
the Almighty Power, the Incomprehenſible Wiſdom, and the Infinite
Perfections of the *Deity*.

† *Moufet Inſect* p 200

F I N I S

E R R A T A.
Pag. 7 *l* 15. inſtead of *other ſpinal*, read, *others ſpiral.* *Pag.* 2? *l* 23 inſtead of
Plate VI read, *Plate* XI. *Pag* 25 *l.* 3 inſtead of *Seed*, read, *Seeds* *Pag.* 35 *l* 26.
inſtead of *Fig.* 2. read, *Fig* 4. *Pag.* 48. in the Running-Title, after, *the Gnat*, place
a full Point

I N D E X.

Constituent

INDEX.

L quor,

FINIS.

CPSIA information can be obtained
at www.ICGtesting.com
Printed in the USA
BVHW040838040619
550106BV00010B/279/P

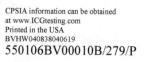

9 781385 562383